WOUNDED

MEN,

BROKEN

PROMISES

ROBERT KLEIN

MACMILLAN PUBLISHING CO., INC.

New York

COLLIER MACMILLAN PUBLISHERS

London

WOUNDED

MEN,

BROKEN

PROMISES

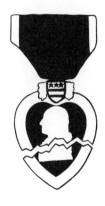

Material from *The Shadow of Blooming Grove,* copyright © 1968 by Francis Russell, is reprinted by permission of The Sterling Lord Agency, Inc. Material from *Mother Jones* magazine and from *Ring the Night Bell* by Paul B. Magnuson, published by Little, Brown and Company, reprinted by permission. Some material in this book originally appeared in the Albuquerque *News.*

Contents

Acknowledgments

My work on this book was made much easier by the dedication and kindness of many people: Patricia Hughes, editor of *Stars and Stripes,* who made her files and thoughts available to me; Lew Milford, of the National Veterans Law Center, who helped put the actions and inactions of the VA into a more comprehensible framework; Gloria Peterson Johnson; Dean Phillips; Jeff Radford, my editor at the *News,* who encouraged me to pursue my original series of articles on the VA and who read portions of the unfinished manuscript; Jack Newfield, who, through his advice about an editor and publisher, was instrumental in making this book possible. My lengthy stays in Washington, a town at once charming and overbearing, were made comfortable and even enjoyable by the boundless hospitality and good cheer of my friends Betsy and David Hawkins. Their home became my "office" and Betsy my inadvertent "secretary," who will not let me forget that Tim Kraft and the White House never returned my calls.

There are several other people without whose help this volume could not have been written. Susan Conway and Robert Levy, two of the world's best lawyers and my close friends, fine-combed the manuscript in detail beyond the call of anyone's duty. Aside from putting the book into clearer focus for me, they were always available in those intimidating hours when I was convinced that I could better serve mankind by digging ditches. For that and many, many other tangibles and intangibles, thanks—and much love.

From Trinidad (Bobby) Padilla, I learned in painful detail about the courage of a maimed Marine as he coped with the war-caused ravages of a torn body. I am also grateful to him for helping me understand the context within which an ex-GI must cope with his government after military service. It was Bobby's idea to include the cracked Purple Heart on the book's cover; the medal, its meaning deeply embedded in his being, is a poignant reminder of what Bobby Padilla has contributed to his nation— and to this book. Linda Mitchell, Bobby's wife and my photographic compadre during my initial newspaper series on the Albuquerque VA, spent long hours transcribing tapes for me. Her concern for all veterans and her vigorous support of my efforts throughout this enterprise were always a source of comfort. Both Bobby and Linda have taught me what it is like to be a wounded veteran, and a concerned citizen, in the United States. I am indebted to them.

Special thanks must go to Ron Bitzer, a whirlwind patient/veteran advocate and tireless VA observer who established my contact lines to people and information when I had just started my research. If it weren't for Ron, who patiently put up with my intrusive week-long visits to his place in Long Beach, this book would have much less merit and interest than whatever it may have now. It is because of Ron and his Center for Veterans Rights in Los Angeles that thousands of veterans across the country, but especially in Southern California, are now much less isolated in their quest for fairness and justice. Ron Bitzer is a magnificent fighter for human rights, and American veterans are lucky to have him on their side. I am proud to be his friend.

Finally, of course, this book could not have been written if I did not receive the unstinting cooperation of many veterans and their families. Because of their pride and a burning desire to see wrongs addressed, they were gracious and open in their long hours of conversation with me—a stranger with a tape recorder and lots of questions. I apologize to the many vets I spoke to whose material was not used in this volume, people like Frank Moore, Barbara Porter, and Bobby and Maria Rodriguez: Be assured that your strength, pain, and convictions sustained me continuously. All of you have shown me that there is, after all, a soul out there in this land of ours. It is to you, and your buddies whom I never met but whose stories I feel I already know, that this book is dedicated.

It is sometimes hard for me to show my appreciation, especially after contending with blank sheets of paper at a variety of ungodly hours in the morning, but it is there, Norma, Lisa, and Andy, it is there. I am grateful for your love and patience. Muchas gracias.

Introduction

This book is about America.

More precisely, it is the story of America's response to thirty million of its citizens and their families whose lives were disrupted, in varying degrees and in varying circumstances, by their nation's continuing call to arms. It is not a particularly complex story, because pain is rather straightforward and uncompromising in its insistence, not unlike the veterans described in these pages. And the issue itself is clear: the lack of consistent, easily obtainable quality medical care—compassionate, meaningful, sensitive treatment—for this country's long line of former servicemen and women.

For the scores of veterans I have interviewed—from Marine officers to Army draftees, from an Arizona postal worker to a Long Island lawyer—the story is an objective retelling of the experiences they encountered as they waded through unrelenting bureaucracy searching for the benefits and respect that had been solemnly promised at the recruiting station. By extension, their report is also about the search for adequate health care for all our people.

A government study notes that the number of hospitals in the United States is decreasing, especially in poor areas. That is no less a crime than is the more directly abusive treatment inside a hospital.

Make no mistake. The Veterans Administration, mandated by Congress in 1930 to provide health care to eligible veterans, is far from monolithic. Many of its consumers, perhaps even a majority, have received, and continue to receive, relatively responsible and responsive medical attention. During my cross-country travels, I met some of the people who, despite overextended case loads and the interference of heavy-handed bureaucrats, still managed to point their faith and energies toward the promotion of quality care at the VA. I am thinking of people like Dr. Paul East and Dean Phillips, both outspoken anomalies in the constricting confines of the Central Office in Washington. I also have in mind Gloria Peterson Johnson, the radiology technician and tireless union president at the Albuquerque VA who, in the face of almost daily obstacles from management, is still able to maintain a vision for her fellow workers and patients alike. And I am talking of Tom Sherwood in New York, a VA administrator who scratches and fights for the sanctity of patient self-respect.

But the calibre of those employees, and their dedication, is not the point. A hospital by definition exists to take care of the sick, the injured, the hurting. Johnson and Sherwood are only fulfilling that mission, that undisputed mandate. The distress, then, surfaces when those who have the power to make things better remain silent. And that does happen, frequently, and it is hard for most of us to believe. It was for me. What I found out made a lasting impression.

It is important to understand what I brought with me to this book. Except for two uncles who spent somewhat uneventful tours in World War II, there is no American military background in my personal life. A participant in the sixties, I escaped the Vietnam War—if any American can be said to have escaped that consuming conflagration. My contact with the war was in the streets: marches on Washington, tear gas on Fifth Avenue, jail.

Hell, no, I didn't go. In 1970, with body bags reaching our shores with obscene regularity, the VA's entire medical budget for the year ($1.6 billion) was less than one month's military expenditures in Vietnam. "We have entered a new marketing era," said the Health Policy Advisory Center, a medical watchdog group, "the age of the disposable GI."

To participate in the war was to acquiesce in American militarism.

So when Robert Shadron walked into my office at the Albuquerque *News* several years ago, my first inclination was to tell the ex-Marine SOB to get lost—or worse. He didn't. Actually, he was downright persistent, and his tale of horror at two VA hospitals—Albuquerque and Houston—ultimately became, for me, a two-and-a-half-year immersion into the workings of the nation's second largest federal agency. (Not coincidentally, the largest is the Department of Defense.) That odyssey permanently changed my view of veterans. They are a hardy lot, most of them drafted away from home and friends, and they deserve better after coming back from a war, or preparations for a war, they didn't make. I came to be particularly impressed with their stamina and surprising good will. Many veterans I met were sick and in pain, but they preserved a faith in their country that was startling. They had fought for their country, they said, and their country would not now let them down.

While my views toward veterans changed, my views about their role in America did not. My experiences just confirmed the perception that veterans, like numbers of their countrymen and women, had been used, only to return home to find themselves discarded by their government like so many spent bullets on the fields of battle. I also discovered, as I had already strongly suspected, that this "throw-away" attitude was not limited to the current generation of soldiers, although it was by and large its courage and anger—and loudly articulated recognition of deceit —which first aroused the public's interest. Of the contributions made by the Vietnam combatant to this nation, from the dead soldier to the live veteran, surely the raising of our collective consciousness must be placed at the top.

In truth, Shadron's story was not my first contact with the VA.

As an aspiring psychologist, I had spent brief periods of time in the early sixties as a trainee at the Gulfport, Mississippi, VA and the Asheville, North Carolina, VA. My strongest memory of the experience was a visit to Gulfport one weekend by a black VA Chief Psychologist. I was nearly lynched by University of Mississippi medical students because I dared to befriend the man. And while I am not exactly a complete novice when it comes to the VA, many Americans are. I especially think of the 18- and 19-year-olds who now must register with the Selective Service system. Do they know what their possible entry into the military means, and what their discharge from it promises? The VA is part of that package. For some, it's the bait—free medical care, education, maybe a car —that guarantees a signature on the dotted line. It is also, for many, the sweet talk that turns sour in the throat.

Experiences with the VA have served to further radicalize an already radicalized generation. Many Vietnam veterans came back from the war with more pronounced leftist leanings than they had when they went in. And not a few older veterans—I have in mind one World War II vet in particular—have told me that because of their own VA experiences, they would sooner their sons go to Canada than fight in the U.S. Armed Forces.

That, I submit, is serious business. What does it mean for the future of the VA? The future of the country? Of the world?

We used to ask, on the streets of the sixties, What if they gave a war and nobody came? That is still a good, pertinent question. But it should be amended to include, What if they promised medical care after the war, and nobody got it? What then?

Current VA practices offer some clues. It is true the VA has been a pioneer in the treatment of spinal cord injuries (though not the unblemished forerunner it would like the public to think). It is true the VA has produced Nobel laureates (with the help of VA patient–subjects). But it is also true that the VA sticks in the craw of millions of America's veterans and their families.

This book may paint a harsh picture of the VA; if so, it is with the hope that some changes will be made, that some dignity will be restored, some treatment improved. The point, finally, is not whether this disturbing chronicle is balanced, for I have uncovered an unpleasant picture of the VA, one that many officials would prefer to keep hidden in the bowels of the bureaucracy. I have shown a side that hasn't been shown.

How else can we be fair to our fellow citizens who have expected, and deserved, more from the Veterans Administration, from their country? "It's time to straighten some of this stuff out," a veteran dying from Agent Orange poisoning told me one very hot summer day in rural North Carolina. He was too weak to move, and he had to be fed by his wife.

"You know what I mean?" he asked me hopefully.

Yes, I know what he means.

Albuquerque, New Mexico
November 1980

Remember that this is a Democratic administration and we are open to all. There are no "dirty tricks" to hide.

—Marthena Cowart, Staff Assistant
to VA Administrator Max Cleland

For it's Tommy this, an' Tommy
   that, an' "Chuck him out, the
   brute!"
But it's "Saviour of 'is country,"
   when the guns begin to shoot;
Yes it's Tommy this, an' Tommy
   that, an' anything you please;
But Tommy ain't a bloomin' fool
   —you bet that Tommy sees!

—Rudyard Kipling

WOUNDED

MEN,

BROKEN

PROMISES

To care for him who shall have borne the battle,
and for his widow, and his orphan.
                    —*Credo on all VA stationery*

I

WAR AND PEACE

The least of Trinidad Padilla's problems with the Veterans Administration is that some half dozen pages of his presumably locked confidential medical files at the Albuquerque VA Medical Center have what appear to be large tire tracks on them.

"It looks like a truck ran over the thing," Padilla, twenty-nine, says. "I don't know if someone took my folder home for nighttime reading, or what."

The husky former marine sergeant has been unemployed since his combat duty abruptly ended in Danang, Vietnam, after eighteen months on February 5, 1970, when a booby-trap grenade exploded three feet away from him and slammed him against the stump of a nearby tree. The shattering blast left Padilla permanently disabled, with slivers of shrapnel embedded deep in several parts of his lower torso. It also left him with a pronounced limp, a sturdy wooden cane, and lots of pain.

Ever since, he has been in and out of the VA hospital, seeking treatment that would enable him to resume a semblance of the active life he had before being shipped, via an honor platoon at Camp Pendleton, to Southeast Asia.

So far he has failed.

Two years ago, Padilla, from the small cattle and railroad town of Belen, twenty-five miles south of Albuquerque, requested and obtained his medical record and examined its contents at length for the first time. The file was eight inches thick. Aside from the apparent tire marks, what Padilla found inside its worn covers horrified him, producing almost as much anguish as the grenade fragments that the VA refuses to concede are still lodged in his left hip.

"I had a piece of shrapnel in my leg when I was discharged," Padilla says. "In fact, I had shrapnel all over my body from the grenade. When I was admitted to the hospital during my last stay, the doctors told me the metal in my hip was too small and too dangerous for surgery, that it might do more damage than good if it was operated on. I was told more or less to go home and suffer."

This conversation, Padilla contends, was never inserted into his chart, nor were other critical pieces of information. "Whatever doesn't suit them gets lost. That's why I was so upset when I finally got my folder. I really don't trust them."

Even material in the chart is ignored.

In his radiographic report of December 27, 1977, the attending physician states that x-ray films of Padilla's left hip reveal "a small subcutaneous foreign body . . . anterior to the upper part of the femoral shaft."

"That," insists Padilla, "is where I've been telling them I've had pain that you wouldn't believe."

Progress notes dated the same day indicate that there is a "foreign body in the soft tissue" in the hip area. A consultation sheet, also on the same date and prepared by an unidentified staff person (a violation of VA regulations), states under provisional diagnosis, ". . . retained foreign body. . . ." The progress note for the clinical case conference on January 18, 1978, reads, "He [Padilla] is having severe pain in his left hip (shrapnel remains)." The note is signed by two psychiatrists, including the chief, Psychiatry Service.

Padilla's hospital discharge summary, written by an orthopedic resident still in training and nominally under supervision, states flatly that Padilla was admitted for "evaluation of chronic pain in the left hip and left thigh which is not related to any trauma. The patient reports the de novo [new] onset of this pain four or five months ago and can cite absolutely no reason whatsoever for the appearance of this pain. . . . The patient tends to relate the pain to old shrapnel injuries in the distal portion of the same leg."

"I don't know what they teach them at medical school," Padilla says bitterly, "but it sure isn't how to read a chart."

Because that report, which was not read or approved by the resident's supervisor as required, denies the existence of shrapnel, despite the VA's own physical evidence, Padilla was ineligible for the increased disability payments afforded veterans when they are hospitalized for more than twenty-one days. Padilla, in the hospital nine weeks, also cannot receive any monthly compensation for the war-connected pain. And, most important, the pain is still there.

"They said it's not service-connected. The doctor told me he would see that I didn't get any disability money for my stay in the hospital. He said he was tired of veterans stealing from the government," Padilla recalls. "All that time I was treated very poorly and very sarcastically by him. He said he'd boot me out of the hospital."

Years before, the suffering had already turned unbearable when, to no avail, Padilla approached the VA for help. His trips to the health facility at the southern edge of the city produced no relief from the extreme discomfort. Doctors said then they doubted the existence of any physical cause of the pain. So, following a well-established pattern familiar to many veterans, they began to schedule psychiatric consultations and counseling for Padilla, who was willing to try anything that might alleviate the consuming hurt.

"They're indifferent, you know," Padilla says. "If you complain or if they can't figure out what's wrong, they'll come up and say you have to see a psychiatrist. They think it'll intimidate you."

Padilla's November 8, 1972, hospital summary piously characterizes his problems as stemming from an "adjustment reaction to adult life, severe, with paranoid and depressive features." The note, with its permanent stigmatization, fails to address the unintended irony of the psychiatric phraseology. Nor does it add that the symptoms implicit in the statement—extreme suspicion, nightmares, suicidal tendencies—are found with frightening frequency in a great many of the men who returned home after fighting in Indochina—something the VA acknowledged as early as 1971 but didn't get around to doing anything about until October 1, 1979.

Because there were no official labels at the time appropriate to what the returning veterans had experienced (the American Psychiatric Association finally came up with one—posttrauma stress —in 1979), Padilla and his suffering comrades had to contend with mental health workers trying to readjust their patients' reactions to adult life, which in this case was nothing more serious than the aftereffects of killing, seeing your close friends blown up, and then being called murderers by your neighborhood pals—and, for some, having to cope with fierce but unacknowledged physical and emotional pain as well.

"I saw I had a nervous condition," Padilla says, "but only because of my wounds, not because I'm psychotic."

Disconsolate at the lack of progress he was making, unable to maintain a job or complete his college courses because of the "stabbing, ripping" agony, Padilla was reading a magazine one day when he noticed a story about an electronic medical device used for the reduction of pain. Until then his treatment consisted mainly of periods of time in the Hubbard tank, a whirlpool-like apparatus.

Though his doctors at first expressed only vague interest in the machine, and tried to talk him out of requesting it ("It costs too much," they said), Padilla persisted and the device was ordered. Padilla, after months of usage, says, "It helps, but it doesn't take away all the pain."

On the horns of a dilemma not of his own making, other than having voluntarily enlisted in the Marine Corps and getting shot up in Vietnam, Padilla cannot work and he cannot get increased service-connected compensation for the grenade attack.

Strangely, the electronic pain reducer that Padilla insisted on getting was made available to him as service-connected treatment for the pain—at the same time the VA was denying any physical source of the anguish.

"There are," says Padilla, who claims to have the distinction of having been spat upon by Jane Fonda as he walked past a 1968 California antiwar demonstration in his marine dress blues, "contradictions throughout the record." It is these contradictions, he says, that deprive him of the benefits he needs to survive and that portray him as less than deserving. The contradictions also raise the question, Who is responsible for a veteran's treatment at the VA?

For instance, Padilla points out, the orthopedic resident wrote in his discharge summary that the "patient [Padilla] was maintained on absolute bedrest for about three weeks and did not adapt to this regimen well, persisting in getting up for any of a number of reasons. He was allowed up for bathroom privileges but was frequently seen out of bed." Later, his summary concludes, ". . . he seemed to have no ambition whatsoever to be discharged. . . . He seemed quite content to spend hour after hour lying around in his bed or in a bedside chair reading books and watching TV." He also said Padilla was depressed. Elsewhere, he says that Padilla can be fully employed.

Aside from the basic incompatibility of the two summary paragraphs—persistence in getting up versus hours of lying around in bed, for example—there are other considerations that were lacking in the chart. According to the widely used *Textbook of Medicine,* "Chronic pain is both physically debilitating and psychologically demoralizing. . . . Psychogenic [psychological or mental] factors always play a role in chronic pain—the pain is more severe when the patient is anxious and stressed and less severe when he is relaxed. The physician must assess the psychologic factors in any patient with pain."

Padilla says his records, when he saw them, were incomplete and not in any kind of order. They contained, he claims, misstatements of facts and misrepresentations, and entire portions of his medical history were missing.

The problem apparently is systemwide. VA Circular 10-79-58,

an in-house memo from the Deputy Chief Medical Director and not for general public circulation, dated March 22, 1979, warns, under Medical Records, "Management at all Medical Centers should review their controls to assure appropriate documentation and timely processing of medical records." And, referring to the chronic related problem of lost or misplaced charts, the circular reminds VA staff, "Failure to release medical information in a timely manner can result in delay of benefits to veterans, and cause adverse publicity for the agency or penalties under the Privacy Act."

Robert Alvarez, chief, Medical Records, at Albuquerque, says that some twenty-five charts are missing at any one time, out of thousands used each month. "No system is perfect. I'm sure some records are lost through the years. Some patients walk home with them or patients don't bother to bring them back." Other workers suggest that overburdened doctors bury charts under piles of other paperwork, and that that accounts for some of the missing charts.

"What they've done to me they've done to other veterans, too," Padilla suggests. "I want to stress the fact that no matter what my physical complaint, I was treated badly. You don't expect everyone to kiss your butt, but, dammit, you have medals, an honorable discharge, and then you come out here and get treated like this."

Angry and frustrated, Padilla took advantage of a public offer from the VA for dissatisfied veterans to call Al Washko, the hospital's assistant administrator. Two days after submitting a list of complaints, Padilla went to speak with Dr. T., chief, Orthopedics Department, and the orthopedic resident's supervisor. Acknowledging some of Padilla's concerns, Dr. T. made several changes in the discharge summary, though Padilla was far from completely satisfied.

Dr. T. later admitted that altering a report after a patient has been discharged is "not commonly done," especially if the doctor making the changes is not the same one who wrote the report in the first place. But Padilla thinks charts must be corrected. "How many other veterans have all sorts of mistakes and wrong information in their records? Veterans' lives are affected by what's in those records. What happens when it's biased or distorted information?"

As head of orthopedics, Dr. T., who did not consult the resident, said, "I am responsible for what's written so I suppose I can change it." Even though he is obligated to, he rarely reads resident doctors' reports before a patient leaves, he added. "They're not even typed yet." Padilla's was one of those untyped, unread reports.

Various VA regulations spell out the importance of the supervisory relationship, including the need to maintain current, accurate records and discharge summaries. The regulations, as well as long-standing Joint Commission on Accreditation of Hospitals requirements, indicate the necessity for supervisor signatures as well as identifying the postgraduate year of the resident on progress and discharge notes.

Abuses of this policy are rampant, as suggested by a VA inspector general's investigation into allegations of surgical mismanagement at the NYU Medical School–affiliated Manhattan VA Medical Center. "All groups of new residents [should] be counseled relative to the importance of timely and accurate record keeping," the inspector general recommended.

Despite all the memos and warnings, the problem continues at places like Albuquerque. "The results of our audit . . . ," states a May 19, 1980, VA report on the Albuquerque facility, "show that serious deficiencies still exist relative to documentation of patient care. . . . It is apparent that increased top level direction is needed to ensure that the medical record deficiencies . . . are corrected."

Padilla's resident, who saw active duty in Vietnam, had his own concerns, however. Already in the advanced stages of his residency, he alluded to Padilla's psychiatric diagnosis and alleged personality traits, clearly calling into question the accuracy of Padilla's statements. Then, off the record, he said, "I made a mistake. I guess I should apologize to Padilla, but if the medical school finds out, I could get into trouble. I've spent a lot of time and effort getting this far. It could ruin my career."

"Any organization or place of business gets complaints. Even

Sears gets some complaints, but it's one of the best stores around,"
insists Assistant Administrator Washko. "You always have people
who want to abuse their benefits. That's human nature, to want
more than they're entitled to. Cheating on income tax, it's the
same thing."

Joseph Birmingham, the hospital's director, and a VA employee for more than thirty years, refrains from comparing his
health-care facility with a business that sells men's socks on lay-
away. Instead, he says gravely, "The complaints a veteran has
may be something we are unable to do a damn thing about. Physicians are not gods. They can't wave a wand and cure something.
And I can see how a veteran may be unhappy because of that. But
there simply may not be an answer for these people. Sure there
may be thirty-six, fifty veterans who are dissatisfied. But if somebody says he can't get to talk to somebody here about his problem,
I just don't believe him."

Told that Padilla says he has tried for the past eight years, the
director said, "We shouldn't be dwelling on the past. The question
is, Are we doing the job or not? I can't answer for what might have
happened years ago. If the veterans write to me with a specific
complaint, I'll give them a written response. I think that's being
pretty damn responsive. I think I'm being responsive. And if other
people don't think so, let them prove it."

"I got no consideration at that VA," says Walter Stimson as he
removes something from his back pocket. It is a small gray piece
of stiff paper with faded brown ink, which Stimson keeps safely
nestled in his thin leather wallet, right alongside the official certificate that identifies him as a licensed steam engineer.

Because of its age, Stimson usually keeps his draft card
wrapped in plastic. "That way it stays protected," he says. "I'm
proud of that thing."

Like the engineer certificate, the military ID is obsolete. It is
dated June 1917.

"I didn't tear up no draft card when I went in," he says. "I'm
a proud American—put it that way."

Stimson, born March 5, 1895, in Corbin, Kentucky, "where Colonel Sanders was," is now visited with cataracts, no teeth, no appendix, no gallbladder, and virtually no stomach. He was a soldier from 1918 to 1919 with the American Expeditionary Forces in Siberia. "I was there. It was hell over in Russia. Seventy-two below and you couldn't stand up outdoors. Ought to have been where I was at. It was rough. I mean it was rough."

Stimson turns and places the wallet on the dresser next to his bed. The small bedroom he shares with his wife of fifty-three years in a tidy middle-class neighborhood is more hospital than residence. Medical equipment is everywhere.

Lying on the bed are two green, torpedo-shaped oxygen tanks. An emergency tank stands nearby, ready to be used in the event an emphysema attack requires extra resources. Looking down on the lifesaving machinery from one wall is a large framed picture of a dreamy-eyed Jesus Christ. It hangs above a mirror poised over the medicine-cluttered dresser. On the adjacent wall, a framed U.S. Air Force "Certificate of Service" advises that Stimson once served his country for fifteen years as a heavy-duty maintenance mechanic at Tinker AFB. It is signed by Gen. T. P. Gerrity.

That was after his army hitch.

"I went and didn't ask no questions. I didn't even know where I was going. I went and I came back."

He stops, and his clear eyes draw a blank. With the aid of his heavy wooden cane, he starts to shuffle back into the living room. "Why didn't I get no consideration up there at the VA?" he suddenly, quietly, asks. "Why?"

Stimson spent one month during the winter of 1978 at the VA Medical Center in Albuquerque for his emphysema problems.

"I've never got such brutal treatment as I did at the hospital out here. I couldn't get those canvas straps off. There's no way in God's world could you get it off if you had to."

Stimson was tied to his chair with Posey restraints, which fastened in back where he couldn't reach them. With no one else in the room, he was kept that way so he couldn't get back into bed to lie down and rest. "They locked the wheels on my wheelchair," he continues. "Left me alone all day. I sat there until suppertime and they'd come back and say, 'You gettin' tired, old man? You'll eat when we get through with you.'

"They put the urine and water bottle where I couldn't reach it. Then they got me up one hour before the others got up and cleaned me before the doctor got there. As soon as he left, they'd tie me up and start that stuff again.

"But I didn't die. Something kept me here.

"The doctor, he's one fine doctor. He takes time to tell you what's wrong. You know, most doctors won't take the time to talk to you. But he spent the time to do it. But the others—they come as near to killing me—well, I never think I've been that close to death. I think they killed me once, I really do. Those big goons supposed to be nurses' aides were just bouncers, that's all. They watch TV and sat around and made fun of me. I'll swear by God and man they did it.

"That hospital management, something has to be done about it, something has to be done about it."

Stimson takes a breath. For a moment it appears as if he might need the oxygen lying in wait a few steps away. His frail frame, down to less than 100 pounds from the 127 he weighed only weeks earlier, seems to disappear into the gray knit shirt holding his skin and bones in place. But the shallow breathing is not from the emphysema.

Instead, Walter Stimson begins to cry. He looks down at the yellow slippers on his feet. "I was a rugged duck," he says softly. "I was operated on in a general hospital in San Francisco. There was no VA then. I had the flu in Vladivostok. Now they threaten to take my pension away from me. I was an oilfield driller for fifty years. I battled oilfield fires and all that stuff. Don't you think a man of my caliber is entitled to more, to decent treatment? They wouldn't give me nothing.

"They say what's the matter with that man? 'Oh, he's crazy.' They didn't say that when I went to Russia. No, they didn't. It froze up for forty miles out to sea. Had to bring us in with dogsleds. I didn't have a care in the world then. I got an honorable discharge. Wasn't too much on it, but I was there just the same."

Across the room, on top of the big color TV console, is a color photo of the Stimsons' fiftieth wedding anniversary celebration. The wall behind is covered with the likenesses of eleven grand-children and nineteen great-grandchildren. One of the figures in the photos is Myra Evans, Stimson's daughter. She is a licensed practical nurse, and she, too, spent a month at the same VA hospital her father stayed in.

"I've been a nurse since 1966," she says, "and I never saw anything worse than the way it is there. It's just awful." Her eighty-four-year-old father, she says, was always very tired when she came to visit him. She would remove the restraints and put him back in bed.

"He was in a room all by himself, all day. It made me so mad. It's not right. He's still a human being and shouldn't be treated that way. The men were treated like animals. I'd come home at night and cry."

Evans's experience working in the long-term treatment section only confirmed what she saw her father going through. After four weeks she quit. "One of the other nurses said to me about my patient, 'Oh, don't worry about him. Just hope he lives through your shift.' That's the attitude they have—make sure he doesn't die on your shift. That hospital—it's a sore spot with me."

"You know," says Stimson, "when I came back from Siberia— I was overseas all but six weeks—there was no such thing as the VA. It was the War Department. We put up a battle for the first VA hospital in the United States. It might have been a bad thing we done. Well, we got 'em, and look what we got."

Suddenly, Stimson gets up, goes over to a corner of the room and returns with his hands full. He has raided his treasure of World War I photos, tinted reminders, hundreds of them, of his time abroad, of his comrades-in-arms. Some are faded beyond recognition, but most are reasonably sharp and clear. Many are sixty years old. The monochromatic streets of a just barely post-tsarist Russia, filled with foreign troops and a newly arisen political conceit, bring smiles to Stimson's face.

"I served my country, and I served it well. But I'll die flat on my back on this floor before I go back to that hospital." He glances up from a crisp photo of himself—a young, bold man in uniform standing in front of a crowded railroad station. "As far as I'm concerned, they treated me like a dog."

Raymond "John" Jones still cannot bathe himself, and bringing a fork to his mouth still requires a great deal of physical effort. But the sixty-one-year-old World War II combat veteran, a former machine-gun infantryman under General Stilwell in the South Pacific, is now able to walk with the aid of parallel bars, and he can once again dress himself.

Two and a half years ago, after he had suffered a series of strokes, his wife brought him to the local VA hospital. She was told to leave him there to die.

"The doctor at the VA pulled me aside," Francine Jones recalls. "He said, 'You have a very sick husband.' I said, 'I know that.' He said, 'The only thing we can do is keep him here and when he dies we'll call you.' I said, 'I took care of him at home before, I'll do it again.' They said they would take him off my hands. I went outside, put my head down on the side of the curb, and cried like my heart would break. And then I went inside and took him home."

Francine Jones smiles faintly at the retelling and wipes her eyes. Responding to a signal, she walks across the living room of their rented home in the valley and attends to her husband of thirty-seven years. Gently, she lowers the huge recliner that serves as bed and chair, leaves his side momentarily, and returns with an empty green plastic pitcher. To the left of where Jones is lying, a gun rack filled with rifles and pistols stands against the wall.

"When I told John I was taking him to the VA hospital, he started crying. He thought he was going to have to stay there," Mrs. Jones, fifty-five, says. "If the veterans' hospital agreed to sign him in and let me sit right next to him and let me be there to see every medication they gave him and everything they did to him, then maybe they could keep him there for three or four days. But to sign him in and leave him there alone—there's just no way I'd do that."

Mrs. Jones leans over and takes the plastic pitcher, now filled with urine, from her husband, rearranges the recliner to its up-right position, and briefly disappears. "People told me to get the veterans' hospital to help," she says, returning to the worn, stuffed seat opposite the recliner. "They said, 'He's a vet, the VA can help.' So I took him to the emergency room. He sat there, or, rather, he lay there, for four hours. Remember, he just had another stroke.

"Finally, my brother-in-law got somebody by the nape of the neck and demanded a doctor, or somebody, see him. The doctor wouldn't touch him. He said he had to be admitted in order to get help. I told him all I wanted was some help at home, I didn't want him to stay in the hospital. I told that to the woman at the VA when I called to ask what to do. I told her all I wanted was some-body to come out and help take care of my husband. The VA does that, you know. They have people who visit the home and help with the care.

"I told her I didn't want the VA's money. I wanted therapy, not money."

Twenty years ago, John Jones—wounded in action, hospital-ized in the Philippines and on Okinawa when the peace treaty was signed—spent five weeks at the same VA hospital for treat-ment of jungle fungus acquired in service. "Nobody knew what was wrong with him," Mrs. Jones remembers. "He came out in worse shape than when he went in. I took him to a private doctor who gave him some ointment. That helped, but the VA didn't do anything."

Now the Joneses, after two decades, are seeking help again. They are convinced that his present problems, significantly more serious than jungle fungus, are in fact service-connected, thereby making Jones eligible for comprehensive VA benefits. Under the circumstances, however, their financial situation entitles him to treatment regardless of the origin of the ailment, according to the VA's own regulations.

"What gets me so mad," says Mrs. Jones, "is that he gave five years of his life to serve his country. Now his country is not help-ing him. It really gets to me because we're not asking for a dis-ability check or holding our hands out for money. You'd think I was trying to take gold out of their filled teeth. But I don't want their money. Let them keep it in Washington to line their pockets. All I want is some help for my husband before he dies."

Mrs. Jones contacted a local neurologist, who had John Jones immediately admitted to a private hospital. Within two weeks the man the VA offered to let die on its wards was walking with the aid of parallel bars. And he was dressing himself, having been guided by the staff at the private hospital to cope with the aftereffects of his paralyzing strokes.

"The therapist and nurses at the private hospital are the most wonderful people in the world," Mrs. Jones says. "They were so caring, so warm and understanding. They were as excited as I was when he walked." But the bills continued to mount. They had to sell their home. Their church, pastor, and neighbors have seen to it that there is food on the table. And, still unable to move the government, Jones is at home receiving from the private hospital's home health care services the occupational and physical therapy and nursing care his wife had requested from the VA.

They are determined to find the necessary money to keep him alive.

"The insurance pays eighty percent and God pays the rest," says Mrs. Jones. "It's through God's grace that we somehow manage."

And there is something else.

The Joneses have one son buried at the Santa Fe National Cemetery, laid to rest in his blue air force uniform while his pregnant wife sobbed over the trim gravesite.

Another boy has spent thirteen years in the First Air Cavalry. "My son joined the army when he was eighteen," his mother says. "He said if it was good enough for his dad, it's good enough for him. But it wasn't good enough for his dad. I wouldn't let another son of mine go into the service, not with the way they've treated my husband. I just wouldn't. If I had another son, I'd ship him to Canada to keep him from putting on the uniform."

Mrs. Jones also suggests it's time people knew where their money is going. "It's sure not helping the veterans. It's sure not helping John. The VA isn't helping the veteran.

"I'm not asking for the government's money. All I want is

somebody out here to help me with him—a wheelchair, handrails for the bathtub, a therapist once or twice a week, prescriptions filled at the VA hospital. Is that too much to ask for someone who has served his country?"

When Anthony Gonzales was released in mid-1978 from the locked section at the VA Medical Center in Albuquerque, he should have been a happy man. Gonzales, twenty-nine, had never been in a psychiatric facility in his life, and the experience of a two-week confinement left him shaken. It also left him without the treatment he was seeking—for his war-torn left leg.

"There are some strange-acting people here," he says, seated at a small table near his bed on the evening of his fourth day in the hospital. Around him, men of all ages and some of indeterminate age slowly and silently tend to their predinner chores, pretty much indistinguishable, the father of one Korean veteran patient later says, from the routine shuffling at other times of the treatment day.

A younger man, dressed in disheveled lime green hospital-issue pajamas and a bit more clear-eyed than the others, sidles over and motions for a match.

No hospital staff is present.

"They're all tranqued out [tranquilized] like zombies," Gonzales, from a small town in northern New Mexico, says. "They want to give me all those drugs, but I won't let them. I'm not interested in sleepwalking like those guys."

Gonzales politely tells the man in the pajamas he has no matches. The man methodically walks away, looking for someone who does.

Admitted because of extreme depression—at least one record on the ward labeled him a "suicidal personality"—Gonzales claims he was given several doses of Thorazine, a powerful tranquilizer, despite his stated wishes to the contrary and drug company guidelines that recommend its use for psychosis only. "I told them I wanted something for my leg, that's what I need," he says.

Instead, they gave him something for his head and closed the door behind him.

"They ended up putting me in this little room by myself, locked and everything. It was like being in jail. They were trying to make me feel like it was my fault or I was guilty of something. I'm not a criminal. I was never guilty of anything, except trying to get treatment. They haven't done nothing for me, man, nothing— except make me wind up here."

There was a time when the short, copper-skinned Vietnam veteran, an infantryman who stepped on a land mine while on patrol thirty miles south of Qu Lai, begged to be admitted for medical care. The February 1971 blast blew out his left knee and foot, leaving him permanently crippled. "It's amazing," he says evenly from his corner bed in the empty multipatient ward, displaying the emaciated flesh left by the wound. "When I desperately needed to be in the hospital, they wouldn't admit me. Now, when I shouldn't be here, they lock me up."

Gonzales was establishing himself as a well-paid custom gunsmith in Los Angeles, working for a major firm in the field, when in January 1978 his injured leg began to hurt. It had been several years since he was outfitted by the Albuquerque VA for his prosthesis, a sturdy long-legged brace, and the worn device was in apparent need of replacement.

Contacting the Long Beach, California, VA, Gonzales was told that before any action could be taken, officials at the hospital would first have to send for his records in Albuquerque. In March, when they still had not arrived, his boss, concerned about possibly losing a good employee, called Long Beach asking for help for Gonzales. "I didn't get very much information," reports Gonzales's gunsmith supervisor. "Nobody seemed to want to help him down there."

By April, no longer able to work because of the pain and discomfort, Gonzales abruptly left for Albuquerque seeking aid. Hitchhiking to New Mexico, now without an income, and no travel money from the VA, Gonzales was refused in-patient status when he arrived tired and drained at the hospital. He says he was told he could not be admitted without a doctor's request.

Ultimately, after returning home to Raton because he had nowhere to stay in Albuquerque, Gonzales was given an appointment with the VA brace shop in mid-June—six months after first requesting help. Back in Albuquerque for his scheduled evaluation, he was again refused admission to the hospital. By then the pain was unbearable, but he did get to see the head of the facility's orthopedics department—the same man who rewrote Trinidad Padilla's record.

"Dr. T. did say something was wrong with my leg, that I was in no condition to work," recalls Gonzales, "but he still couldn't let me into the hospital. According to him, it wasn't serious enough. One problem, he said, was that I shouldn't be wearing ordinary street shoes. I was never told in seven years that I wasn't supposed to wear street shoes.

"T. wouldn't sign the work order for new shoes and he said he couldn't put me in the hospital, either. I wanted to get taken care of and get back to work. I said, 'Okay, forget it,' and I started to walk off. By that time I was mad, tired, fed up. What can I say?

"And he stopped me, like he was doing me a big favor—and he let me in. The resident physician [assigned to Gonzales—and Padilla] asked me every day when I was leaving. I'd tell him, 'When you fix my leg.' They didn't come in my room anymore. They didn't like to hear that.

"They finally measured me for a new brace and shoes, and sent it off to New York to be made. I told them before they ordered it that it wouldn't fit. My foot's almost gone, there's been so much shot out of it. I knew what would fit and what wouldn't. I've had the problem for seven years.

"When the brace got back, it didn't fit. I knew it wouldn't. They just wasted a pair of shoes, and all that money. They said since it doesn't fit, they wanted to cut my foot to fit the shoe. I told them, 'You don't cut my foot to fit the shoe, you cut the leather to fit my foot.' I said, 'I don't want to do anything drastic, I want to see if the brace works.'"

VA officials, including a top administrator sent specifically to look into the situation at Albuquerque, deny any such suggestion was offered. "That's ridiculous," insists Dr. Robert Love, at the time director of the VA's central office of Operations, Review and Analysis, adding without a trace of irony that "surgery was specifically considered by a team of physicians and decided that it would not be the best course of treatment for Mr. Gonzales."

Dr. T. said he did not know how long it usually takes for a brace to be made. "If it's not finished, it's not finished. I wish they were made quickly. If one person has to wait a couple of months, I suppose there are a lot of people who have to wait a couple of months." Dr. Love called it a "bureaucratic delay that certainly should have been avoided."

Then, warning that the facts should be checked carefully, T. said that not everything that transpires between a physician and his patient is written into the patient's record. "Sometimes we don't like to put things in a chart which we think might get a patient upset," he said cryptically. "Not everything is in writing."

He did not elaborate.

In June, Gonzales was sent to Dallas, at VA expense, for another fitting. He says he spent forty-five minutes being measured, and then got back on the plane to Albuquerque.

"The pain was killing me and I had no job and they didn't know when they would get the shoes from Dallas. I stopped taking all those drugs. They were making me dingey. They kept telling me it's supposed to hurt—if you get wounded, it's supposed to hurt. But they didn't say why.

"I wanted to go back to work. I had to leave my job because of the VA. My boss wants me back, but not unless the VA can do something about my leg. My tools are still there. Having to leave has really brought me down. I wanted to work. I wanted to build up my reputation. I didn't ask to be drafted, or to be in the infantry. But I went. I didn't split. I went unwillingly to fight a country I didn't like. Now I'm ready to fight a country I do like, that's the way I look at it."

With no money, no brace, and no job, and in extreme anguish, Gonzales hitchhiked around the state looking for work while he waited for the vital piece of equipment. It was well into the heat of summer now. "A lot of places were ready to hire me," he says, "until I told them about my leg. I don't blame them for not wanting a man in my condition."

On a Tuesday, July 25, Tony Gonzales returned to the VA hospital, desperately in pain, to inquire about the leg brace measured and ordered over a month before. He had come full circle, begging again for help, for consideration. They told him they still could not be of assistance, that the brace had not arrived, and that they did not know when it would arrive.

So, Tony Gonzales, young and tired and despairing, collapsed emotionally in front of the doctors who said they couldn't help. This time, he was admitted to the hospital—to the psychiatric ward for fifteen days.

"I just really fell apart," he says. "I was all broken up. You couldn't talk to me. I was in pain, man, all over."

Gonzales shakes his head in fury.

"They said they couldn't understand why I got so depressed just because I didn't get my brace."

God and the military veteran, we adore . . .
In times of danger, not before;
The Danger pass'd, and all things righted
God is forgotten and the veteran slighted.
                —*Anonymous World War I soldier*

The VA? Are they still around?
                —*Former Green Beret combat officer*

2

A GENERALIZED MALAISE

Although the 404-bed general medical and surgical facility at Albuquerque is only one of the Veterans Administration's 172 medical centers located in the forty-eight contiguous states, Washington, D.C., and Puerto Rico (Alaska and Hawaii both have out-patient programs only), the problems it projects are endemic, the malaise generalized, the ailment crippling—perhaps fatal.

If the VA were an eligible veteran, it would quickly check into the nearest hospital.

And if it had any sense—or medical insurance—it would choose a non-VA facility for its care.

To be sure, quality varies wildly throughout the nation's largest health-care system, which employed 194, 294 full-time workers and provided in-patient care in 90,154 beds for some 1.3 million veterans in 1978. And, also to be sure, the VA is very much aware that care is not meted out equally everywhere in the agency, which, in addition to the medical centers, includes 220 out-patient clinics, ninety-one nursing-home-care units, eighteen spinal-cord-injury centers, and sixteen domiciliaries (long-term residential-type facilities). And as of October 1, 1979, the VA also began activating the first of its eighty-six informal storefront operations for Vietnam veterans. Annually, the VA provides health care to more than 2.5 million veterans.

But what the VA is loath to make public is a list of just which parts funded by its health-care budget ($5.4 billion in 1979) are better and which worse.

In other words, although a network of monitoring systems is more or less in place, the VA discreetly and adamantly refrains from giving out that information that would enable its consumers —American veterans—to determine just how well, or poorly, they can expect to be treated by any one of the 10,000 physicians, 900 dentists, 28,000 nurses, 22,561 medical residents, 1,398 graduate psychology students, 19,550 medical students, or any of the other tens of thousands of technicians, admitting clerks, and administrators who comprised the agency's medical system in 1978–79. Even though the VA, through its own internal audits as well as from data collected in the massive National Academy of Sciences study released in 1977, knows whether a veteran should go to, say, Albuquerque rather than, say, Long Beach for certain types of medical care, it refuses to release that information.

The health-care system is only one component of the VA. Although it has 90 percent of the employees, it is surpassed in budget by the approximately $10 billion allocated for the legislatively mandated costs of compensation and pension payments to veterans and their dependents. In addition, other benefits read like a veritable smorgasbord of social welfare good works—educational loans, clothing allowances, guide dogs, home loans, special equipment for automobiles, and cemetery burial space with perpetual free care. The VA is also one of the country's largest insurance companies.

In all, there are some seventy-five different benefits programs administered by the VA, making it, in total, second only to the Department of Defense in number of government employees and third among federal agencies in expenditures, with a record 1979 budget of $20.3 billion, just behind HEW. The VA's approximately one-quarter million employees make up a remarkable 8 percent of the federal government's full-time workers. As of September 30, 1978, the VA had spent over $300 billion in total benefits through the years. It is a huge bureaucracy, virtually unknown to the public.

Nonetheless, it is the component of the VA that accounts for slightly more than one-quarter of the entire budget—the Department of Medicine and Surgery—that people identify with the VA. It is a fortuitous coincidence, because how we understand and execute the delivery of medical care to our fellow citizens is a good measure of what—and whom—we value in ourselves. Thus, it is instructive to hear the litany as it echoes from coast to coast, in varying cadences and amplitudes, throughout the system: insensitive management, abrasive staff, abusive care, funding shortages, inadequate facilities, medical school domination, inappropriate staff-patient ratios.

Translated into more personal terms, we hear of malpractice suits, corruption, unnecessary patient deaths, ignored men and women, pain and frustration, angry veterans—and denials by top officials that anything could be significantly wrong with an agency that potentially affects, via the nation's more than 30 million living vets and their families, the lives of virtually one-half the population of the United States.

Disgust with the VA is nationwide, and its expression is often visceral. It is not limited to patient-veteran complaints, either. Nor is it just the malcontented noise of one generation's soldiers. Letters in the March 1979 issue of the magazine of the Disabled American Veterans, an energetic service organization with more than 600,000 members, begin to assess the climate among our wars' comrades.

I have exhausted every remedy except civil action against the VA for severe and irreversible physical and emotional damage. Letters to Congress result in perfunctory, lick-and-a-promise, do-nothing buck-passing. Little Max [Cleland], God love him for his sacrifice and service to our country, but for God's sake, RESIGN! He lacks the vigor, stamina, and the do-or-die spirit to remedy the rapidly deteriorating VA in-patient and out-patient care.

—*Alex H. Wells, Columbus, Georgia*

My husband is a disabled veteran. . . . [Veterans] have served proudly, and now on top of everything, they have to fight and struggle for every inch they win. I think it's a shame that our government wants to forget them so easily.

—*Mrs. Houston Rice, Boswell, Oklahoma*

Why should we be made to feel guilty for being a veteran? We rose to the call of our country in its times of need. . . . Once we were no longer needed to fight and die on the battle front, we have to start a new battle, here at home, to preserve our rights against the same people we served and fought for all those years. It is disgusting!

—*H.N. Parker, Lakeland, Florida*

Elsewhere in the same issue, a report details the conditions found at the Louisville VA by the mother of a totally paralyzed Vietnam veteran who died at the facility. Her son's disability, she said, "had prevented him from taking care of his own needs, . . . he was not given enough water, . . . his meals grew cold at his bedside because he waited as long as an hour for someone to help him eat, and . . . he was cold."

Denying the mother's allegations, hospital administrators skirted the issue, telling reporters the facility "just doesn't have the money to provide the kind of nursing services that private hospitals can provide."

From the May 1979 DAV magazine:

At 75 years of age, I and my wife are fighting for a meager existence. Lost my left eye in line of duty—have been treated for glaucoma by VA and civilian doctors for 10 years. My vision at various times is almost nil. The young doctors here at the VA hospital have taken away my medication and, needless to say, my sight is disappearing rapidly. I shall seek a specialist as soon as possible, and forget the VA. The only word I can add is that the VA has deteriorated.

—*Peter D. Standard, San Diego, California*

Those [Vietnam veterans] I know, if given a chance, would prefer to choose their own medical care, and it would not be at a VA hospital. If you poured all the money in the U.S. Treasury into the VA, it would not change. . . . Dump the mismanaged VA hospital system. . . .

—*Anthony J. Graziano, Somerville, Massachusetts*

And this letter from the October 18, 1979, *Stars and Stripes,* the venerable 104-year-old national veterans' newspaper:

My father was a WW I veteran. I sent him to the VA hospital at Marion, Illinois, on July 23, 1979. They kept him until August 1, 1979, and took away his heart medicine and said there was nothing wrong with him. On August 3, 1979, I had to take him to the Salem Hospital. He was in great pain. They took tests of him and he had to have surgery the same day. He had ulcers and gangrene had set in. They took out half his stomach. He had cancer all through his stomach. He lived until August 14, 1979. What I want to know is, what kind of VA hospital do we have to send our older veterans to when they cannot pay their bills? I am left with his bills and don't have the money to pay them. What I am saying is, you had better have money to pay the doctors because they don't have any at that VA hospital. If they did, they would have found what was wrong with my father.

—*Name Withheld*

VA employees also write letters, like this one in the July 26, 1979, *Stars and Stripes* from a nurse, Jim Dunn, at the Bath, New York, VA facility. The hospital's director, characterized by at least one employee as possessing the psychology of a Captain Queeg, tried to get the VA Central Office to sue the nurse and the union because of the letter's contents. Dunn is a representative of Local 491 of the American Federation of Government Employees.

The biggest loser is the patient, whose misfortune is two-fold. One, his financial position which required him to seek medical help from the VA. His second misfortune is in being admitted to a VA hospital. The patient must be submitted to a de-humanizing process that makes euthanasia look inviting.

A patient is brought to the VA, but cannot get good medical attention. There are many days that go by that a patient doesn't see his doctor. The doctor is running helter-skelter to cover his many floors. The nursing personnel are stretched; . . . Staffing is too short to care for the human whose life they hold. . . . Without the needed interaction of needed hours of mental rehabilitation, once mentally alert individuals become the easy vegetables with which to work. As long as the patient doesn't offer rational interaction, one doesn't feel bad leaving him sit for hours staring at a meaningless TV or silent walls. Let a patient offer rational thinking and there isn't the time to interact anyway. . . .

Or the letter from Rep. Bill Nichols, a member of Congress from the Third District of Alabama, who wrote to an Oklahoma veteran that it "makes me boiling mad to see our veterans receiving second class treatment [at the VA]." Nichols, heavyset and cautious, is a severely wounded World War II veteran with one leg gone and the other paralyzed. "Nothing brave," he says, "just stepped on a mine in Germany in 1944.

"Our VA hospitals, in my judgment, are oftentimes understaffed. I have complaints from veterans who say they often get a nurse or orderly instead of the doctor simply because the staff waits on more patients than they have to," he said in an interview. He says his main concern about the Birmingham VA—the largest in his state—is the waiting time. "It's atrocious. And then when they get to see the doctor, the patient load sort of dictates them being prone to getting a lick and a promise.

"There are some people associated with our veterans' hospitals whose attitudes are not what they're supposed to be," Nichols adds. "A few who take the sort of an attitude—'What are you grumbling about, bitching about, it's free.' That just irritates the hell out of me because those boys have paid the price. They've paid it at Iwo Jima, Salerno, they paid it in the invasion of Normandy, Pork Chop Hill, and they paid it in the delta of Vietnam."

And then there's the letter written on May 6, 1979, by Dr. Gabriel Manasse, a psychiatrist at the VA's Brentwood, California, Day Hospital who was chosen to participate in the VA's program for employees with outstanding leadership and administrative potential. He wrote his letter, he said, "with a sense of urgency inseparable from a sense of impending futility."

The six-page, single-spaced missive was addressed to Mrs. Rosalynn Carter, in care of the White House.

For the first time in my almost seven years at Brentwood, we have had to devise and quite regularly utilize a 'restricted' admitting policy which places non-service-connected veterans who *warrant hospitalization medically* in out-patient programs often *unable* to cope with their needs. . . . Some of the older veterans and staff have been here before—they are used to unfulfilled expectations and unrealized hopes. They will survive and the VA will persist. But America is poorer by far. The very men and women to whom we have such *incalculable* debt—these *I* must face with shame, day in and day out, as I close *my* program door and I am unable to provide services which every clinician and administrator at this hospital knows should be available and to which the veterans are *entitled* . . . *!* It is at this juncture that I must *beg* for your help. . . . The VA, the entire administration, the Congress, indeed ultimately the populace must adopt a new attitude toward its debt to its citizens, especially those poorly able to effectively lobby or otherwise "demand" their due. [Italics in original.]

Dr. Manasse, calling his plea a "long shot," never received a response from Mrs. Carter.

The individual expressions of distress and dismay are bolstered by extensive material. In March 1979 the Disabled American Veterans presented to Congress the results of its survey of the quality of care at VA facilities around the nation. Almost 13,000 questionnaires were returned by DAV members who had recently sought medical treatment from the VA.

The data confirm the deterioration of the VA system: 43 percent said they waited more than an hour before being seen (15 percent waited more than three hours); 37 percent complained of incorrect labeling or late delivery of prescriptions; 21 percent reported discourteous treatment by employees; 91 percent were scheduled for an appointment at the same time as a number of other patients, in direct violation of central office policy. Hospitalized veterans reported similar treatment.

The survey also revealed that some understaffed hospitals have, in part, lost their accreditation—staff-patient ratios are an average of less than two to one, compared with three to one or higher in comparable community hospitals. "Primary nursing is a fantasy here—a paper facade—which can only be done marginally, if at all, with our present staffing," one nurse told the DAV.

Although the VA counters with its own survey statistics, which indicate a far higher rate of favorable attitudes toward VA care, it is still clear that the fury, frustration, and discontent run deep and wide. But the spotted condition of the VA is, like the marching off to war of this country's young people, neither new nor unique.

The VA, in fact, has a long and dishonorable history—older than the official beginnings of the agency itself—replete with cases of widespread scandal, poor and abusive medical care, insufficient funds and inadequate staff, cronyism, questionable legislative authority, delayed implementation of critical medical and other health programs, and, of course, the usual congressional hand-wringing (some say pussyfooting).

Though the present administration—whichever one it happens to be at the moment—would disagree, it is not exaggerating to say that the VA can legitimately point to just one brief moment in its past and honor it with the phrase "a job well done."

Between 1945 and 1947, Gen. Omar Bradley, appointed by President Truman to revitalize a stagnating, abuse-infected VA, headed an agency abuzz with excitement and energy. Bradley told Truman he would stay only two years. Under Bradley the VA saw its zenith. When he left, it tumbled rapidly back into the abyss of bureaucratic insensitivity and sloth.

"Obviously," intones the report of a special Senate subcommittee convened in the late 1940s to assess the post-Bradley disarray, "no medical care program worthy of the name could function on this [badly managed] basis without the rapid development of such confusion, frustration and mismanagement as would quickly wreck morale, drive out competent personnel and rob the program of any possible value to anyone but such selfish incompetents as might be willing to pretend to work in the resulting shambles."

But committee reports do not a viable agency make—not without any follow-up, they don't.

On July 15, 1979, thirty years after the Senate's lament, VA Administrator Max Cleland told a gathering at the national convention of the Disabled American Veterans in Boston, "When I first encountered the VA medical system in 1968 as a patient, my own satisfaction was not high. It was obvious that there was need of improvement in many areas: staff-to-patient ratio was far too low, many facilities were physically unsuitable, specialized medical services were inadequate, and there too often was a lack of concern among the staff. The system was, in essence, not up to the task."

Implicit in his remarks is the assumption that Cleland and his staff, many of them either fellow Georgians and/or former army buddies, have gone far in cleaning up the mess they inherited. In fact, this is not so. Indeed, Cleland, who frequently talks as if the VA has no substantive past—he rarely does more than make a fleeting reference to the post–World War II era—is not ashamed to call the VA "the conscience of the country toward our nation's veterans," as he did in his first official act as administrator when he sent a message of greetings to "my associates in the Veterans Administration."

It is, however, a conscience that charges across the land in headlines and stories that sear the newsprint.

SIX VET-PATIENTS COMMIT SUICIDE AT VA HOSPITAL IN DOWNEY, ILL.
—Veterans' newsletter, November 1975

STAFF SHORTAGES, OVERCROWDING, DIRT AND LEAKY ROOFS IN A MEDICAL SLUM
—Life, *May 22, 1970*

PATIENT FOUND TIED TO HER BED TRIGGERED VA PROBE
—New York Post, *June 16, 1979*

N.J. CHARGES VA HOSPITAL WITH ABUSES
—Hackensack Record, *August 2, 1979*

VA DROWNING TRAGEDY—MISSING LONG BEACH PATIENT'S BODY FOUND IN TUB
Long Beach Independent Press-Telegram,
May 17, 1978

WIFE SUES VA HOSPITAL IN "WRONG MEDICINE" DEATH
Long Beach Independent Press-Telegram,
May 11, 1978

VETERAN OF 34 YEARS UNABLE TO GET HOSPITALIZATION AID
Albuquerque Tribune, *November 30, 1978*

COSMETIC SURGERY AT VA HOSPITAL TOLD
Los Angeles Times, *December 15, 1978*

STAFF DOCTORS CALL SOME VA POLICIES "MEDICAL MALPRACTICE"
Tampa Tribune-Times, *June 24, 1979*

THE VETERAN AS GUINEA PIG
New Times, *November 27, 1978*

DUBIOUS SURGERY REPORTED FOUND IN VA HOSPITAL
New York Times, *October 2, 1979*

VETS JOIN IN SUIT FOR AGENT ORANGE VICTIMS' CLAIMS AGAINST VA
Stars and Stripes, *June 7, 1979*

Vietnam veterans, especially the 300,000 who were wounded out of the 2,796,000 sent to Vietnam (150,000 had to be hospitalized and 75,000 were severely handicapped), have complained long and loud about the quality of treatment they have received (or, in many instances, unsuccessfully tried to receive) from the VA. They have convincingly documented the insensitivity of a government that ignored their needs and concerns once their bullets, and lives, had been spent overseas.

Even Cleland acknowledges the VA has not done all it should for the Vietnam veteran. Still, it is misleading to blame all the troubles on those now in power. Certainly the current administration has placed its own telling mark on the way things are run at the huge agency. But the Vietnam veteran, with the misfortune both of participating in a discredited war and of entering the VA system when the dollars to wage that war were being drained from *all* health-care services, including the VA, is getting dumped on from a load that has accumulated during the greater part of this century. To recognize otherwise is to misunderstand and excuse the de facto role of the VA—and turn our backs on *all* American servicemen and -women, and the nation they served.

"I think the Vietnam veteran has helped the veterans of other wars in terms of highlighting and focusing on what our priorities are in dealing with our veterans," says Dave Christian, the youngest man ever chosen commander of the elite Legion of Valor and the youngest captain to serve in Vietnam. "How should they be handled? Should they get an unjust enrichment? No, but they should be taken care of. They shouldn't have to worry after they've been put under the threat of a gun.

"Veterans had to face those problems from Vietnam all the way back. Vietnam just highlighted it," adds Christian, the holder of a dozen battle awards and the brother of two younger brothers disabled in Vietnam. "The VA should not be considered a drain on society. What it should be doing is taking care of our most valuable resources, our young men, our young women. It should be taking care of them and putting them back together.

"If the government could find us in time of a war and take care of the problems of war, then they could find us and take care of the social problems, the psychological problems, the medical problems in times of peace. We're easy enough to be found.

"We have discarded the veteran. The Veterans Administration is acting like the veteran has become a discarded army. People say, ah, the Vietnam veteran is no good, a deadbeat. But how come he wasn't a deadbeat when he was taken away from his family? How come he wasn't considered a deadbeat when he was trained for a uniform and to shoot a rifle? How come today he is a deadbeat?"

Like a giant *déjà vu* machine, the VA sees generations of returning veterans come and go while the problems and complaints, garbed then in doughboy khaki, dressed now in 'Nam resolve, remain the same. Today, Vietnam veterans speak bitterly of the older VA employee, those men and (some) women who, finished with their duties at the end of the Big War, now block the paths of benefits and rehabilitation due the younger soldier.

"Why does the VA respond that way? It's the little people from the class of '46," suggests Ken Baker, a thirty-three-year-old veteran of two tours in Vietnam who says that if he had a dollar for every vet who avoids the VA, he'd be rich. "The combat vet got all the media attention, but when we got back we were ignored. Vietnam was a bad war. We lost. And the United States couldn't lose. Gotta blame somebody. Not gonna blame Gen. William Westmoreland. Blame us. The old guys in the VA ain't gonna help people like me."

Baker's pain, aggravated by a war-induced disability the VA refuses to acknowledge, is the echo of a plea voiced thirty-five years ago by the very same people—the class of '46 alumni—he now must contend with. Back then, they too demanded consideration from an even earlier class.

"Put the vets themselves in charge of their rehabilitation. Not World War I vets" is the sentiment of a World War II veteran quoted by Charles G. Bolte in his 1946 book *The New Veteran.* "The feeling was widespread," Bolte continues, "that this war's veterans could handle their affairs better than the veterans of the last war, who appeared settled in life."

As if out of the mouth of Baker and his almost three million in-country Vietnam comrades, Bolte writes, "Their recommendations for improvements [in the VA] were headed by the demand that more attention be paid to the individual veteran and his problems; having freshly escaped from the highly institutionalized armed forces, they were not eager to be steered through still more institutional channels. They wanted the runaround ended; they wanted better medical care; and they wanted less delay in the whole process."

"There must be a more efficacious way to help the people who need it most," says Billy Nix, a wounded army Vietnam veteran and assistant supervisor at the DAV office in Atlanta. "Bad service has been going on now since 1930. And it's still going on. But I think it's changing. The younger vets are more loudmouth. It's the times. People aren't afraid to say the government sucks. They may have felt that way in the forties, but they were quiet and didn't say it. The bureaucratic system has just gotten out of hand, period."

"The VA is a system that, at its best, is the best anywhere," says Michael Sklar, Chairman of the Urban Planning Department at Columbia University and formerly an economist with the VA. "At its worst, they should lock up some of the people who work there."

The generations of American servicemen and -women, it is clear, have more in common than spending a part of their lives dodging the mortar and machine gun fire of the enemy-of-the-moment.

"My experience was this. I had to get injections three times a week because my blood pressure wouldn't stay up from the infection I got in the service—from the lye in the food."

It is a hot and muggy September Sunday evening in Los Angeles—the first day of what turned out to be a weeklong pollution alert for the California city—and Jan Roberts is slowly sipping ice water in his cluttered one-bedroom apartment. At sixty-two, Roberts, a World War II veteran and former vice-commander of an LA American Legion post, is an established Westwood tax consultant who once worked for President Truman.

Outside, the hum of air-conditioners cuts through the sagging air. Inside, Roberts sucks on an ice cube and continues his story.

"So, I made arrangements to go to Kingsbridge [VA hospital]. I told them I was trying to work and go to school, finish up my last year. This was just after the war. I would come at seven o'clock in the morning, hoping to get my treatment at eight, which they had agreed to. And I'd end up sitting there until three o'clock in the afternoon and then an orderly, not a doctor, would come in and give me a shot in the arm. He wouldn't even take my blood pressure, my pulse, or anything else. And out the door I'd go.

"One day they were in such a hurry at three o'clock in the afternoon, there were so many people sitting and waiting, and I'd been there since seven—a doctor was supposed to take care of me, not a yard boy—and I saw him give a serum to someone else. And then he turned around and he was going to give me the same thing. I figured there was something wrong. So I asked him, and he caught himself, and he said, 'Oh, no, that's the wrong serum!' But if I hadn't been alert, I would've got the wrong serum. I don't know what kind of damage it would've done.

"I had occasions where needles broke, where they were very careless. I was afraid of reinfection from them. It scared me. I never went back again."

Instead, Roberts, a gruff, outspoken man whose hostility toward injustice has landed him in more than one vat of hot water boiled up by red-faced officials, "in disgust" went to a private physician. "The shots were twenty-five dollars apiece. But I paid it, out of my own pocket." As he did the treatment that he received at a private hospital–medical school for the next ten years.

"My experience with the VA has always been *very bad,*" he says, emphasizing his words.

Even, he recounts, when he is not the patient.

"This young man couldn't use his hands. He was at the Los Angeles VA hospital. It was dinnertime and they brought one of these trays that you push over the bed. And somebody was supposed to come in and feed him."

Roberts was visiting a friend at the time, and noticed the ex-soldier's quiet distress.

"I said to the young man, a Vietnam veteran, 'Would you like me to feed you?' And he said to me, 'It's cold. The food is cold.'

"When he said this, I heard this cackling outside the door of his room. I went outside, into the hall, and this group of orderlies was standing around and just kidding around and playing around, and I said, 'Which one of you men is supposed to come in and feed this poor man?'

"And this kid turns around to me and says, 'Yes, boss, that's me.' I said, *'You son of a bitch.'* I said, 'That kid went over there to fight for you and your rights and your right to live in freedom.' I said, 'And that's how you treat him?'"

Roberts's fury at the retelling is subsiding now. He takes a long, cool swallow of ice water. "So I went back in and I picked up the tray and I handed the orderly the tray and when I did I tilted it right on him. And I said, 'You get your goddamn ass down there in the kitchen, and you bring me back *a hot tray.'*

"It was my purpose to wake him up. And when he brought the tray back—he was in a clean uniform—in the meantime, those other guys got a mop and cleaned up—I took the tray from him and I said, 'I'll feed him.' But I said, 'The next time I find this out, I'm going to come down here and *break your living neck.'*"

Roberts gets up, goes into the kitchen and returns with a full glass of ice cubes and water. He needs to cool off some more. "So this is his infirmity. Because he went off to fight a war he didn't want any part of, they treated him like a pig. Understand? *This I object to.*"

Some sixty minutes south of Jan Roberts, along one of those screaming southern California freeways, Dick Theodore is maintaining his own vigil at home in Garden Grove. Theodore, a construction sheet-metal welder before he fell off a ladder in June 1962 and wound up paralyzed from the waist down, spent three years in the service, from November 1934 through December 29, 1937.

Tonight, he is hosting a meeting of veterans who have had problems with the VA. He is expecting a former VA doctor to drop by. The doctor never shows and Theodore is left to entertain the two veterans who do. "Maybe we can get more accomplished this way," he says.

On the TV, Cronkite is assuring America about FAA inspections and falling DC-10s. Theodore has a remote-control device for turning Cronkite off, but he chooses to leave the CBS news alone. Sitting motionless, his feet in brown cowboy boots, Theodore also has at his fingertips a telephone, a glass of water in a blue plastic glass, pencils, filed VA material, and assorted personal objects— all squeezed together on a gray stand with squeaky rollers. Nearby are two motorized wheelchairs.

At ease in his thick yellow recliner, Theodore's hollow cheeks look hollower, his thin body thinner. He is wearing a Mexican bolo tie, and he urges the few guests to have some Fresca and cookies his wife has brought into the living room.

To one side of the room, a framed photo reveals the smiling image of Theodore resting in one of his motorized wheelchairs. He is relaxed and happy and he is wearing his worn DAV cap at a jaunty angle. Sitting on Dick Theodore's lap is Jane Fonda.

Theodore was one of several veterans who played themselves in brief roles in *Coming Home,* the movie about the Vietnam War that won a specially created media award from the VA, several honors from Hollywood, and lots of questions about the reality of the film's scenes, many of which depicted VA medical care.

Theodore claims the photo of him and Fonda inspired the moviemakers to include a touching moment in which co-star Jon Voight maneuvers his wheelchair while Fonda sits on his lap. "I believe if Jane is given a chance, she'd work for the veteran and be a big help," Theodore says of the experience.

He also thinks the VA hospital scenes, mostly graphic characterizations of despair and lack of care and compassion, were close to the real thing. "The part with Jon [Voight] was a little bit over-done, especially when he was knocking things all over the place," Theodore allows. "If he had done that very much in the hospital, they would have had the straitjacket on him so fast." But, he says, "you take all of your veterans out there, including the ones from Vietnam—that was a pretty accurate movie."

Jan Roberts, back in Los Angeles, is pondering the same verities. Ten years as a Defense Department analyst has only strengthened his attitude toward the veterans' agency.

"The VA is nothing but a big rip-off," he says. "They don't give a damn about the veteran. None whatsoever. They're just there to make the buck. They're hiring the wrong kind of people. There's no feeling for the veteran."

If Jan Roberts's assessment is accurate today, then its genesis must be traced back more than fifty years to July 21, 1930, the day President Herbert Hoover signed Executive Order 5398, officially establishing the Veterans Administration as a separate independent agency. Hoover's signature brought under one administrator all veterans' programs passed by Congress since World War I, and authorized the president to "consolidate and coordinate government activities affecting war veterans."

At the time, there were potentially 4.7 million veterans eligible for benefits from the new bureaucracy's 31,500 employees and fifty-four hospitals. In 1978, 15,069,573 out-patient visits and 1,228,755 hospital patients were listed on VA rolls, the greatest number in the agency's history. Since this country's Revolutionary War and its 290,000 participants, 38,924,000 men and women have served in the armed forces of the United States (over 90 percent in wartime). Fully three-quarters of that number—30 million—are living today, and are eligible for one kind of VA benefit or another.

While two out of every three of these living veterans have in fact used one or more benefits offered by the VA, *less than 15 percent* have *ever* availed themselves of in-patient care. In fiscal year 1978, only 93,053 veterans received care for a service-connected disability—less than 10 percent of hospitalized veterans that year. Similarly, only about 15 percent have ever used the VA's out-patient services. Less than 50 percent of the veterans visiting these clinics go for service-oriented injuries.

(Service-connected injuries are injuries caused or aggravated during an honorably discharged veteran's active time in the service, whether incurred in combat or not. Injuries are rated according to degree of disability—20 percent for loss of a toe, for example; 100 percent for blindness—and appropriate monthly compensation is paid accordingly. In 1978, a 20 percent rating entitled a veteran to $80 per month; total disability entitled the veteran to $809 monthly. Extenuating circumstances, such as combination of losses of bodily parts, or number of dependents, entitle the veteran to additional compensation. The amounts were raised approximately 7 percent in 1979. For a veteran with a family, the limit could rise to some $24,000 a year, tax-free.)

A factor as important as the monetary compensation is a service-connected veteran's priority status for free hospital care. It is he, or she, whom the VA is mandated by law to serve first. Secondary consideration, on a space-available basis, is given to indigent veterans. The overwhelming number of out-patient and in-patient consumers are non-service-connected veterans, although the percentages are changing somewhat owing to an energetic campaign (and budgetary constraints) carried out by Max Cleland to inform the veteran public about the VA's mission. In 1979, for example, use of ambulatory (out-patient) facilities by service-connected veterans increased some 6 to 8 percent within an eight-month span.

Although the VA celebrates its inception from the time of Hoover's penmanship, an accurate and meaningful genealogy would include a potpourri of programs going back to colonial America when, in 1636, the Plymouth Pilgrims adopted a law providing that "if any man shalbee sent forth as a souldier and shall return maimed, hee shalbee maintained competently by the collonie during his life."

Virginia, Maryland, New York, and Rhode Island followed suit, and the Continental Congress in 1776 established pensions for those disabled in battle. Benefits to dependents of American Revolution veterans were paid as late as 1911. Until 1811, most direct medical and hospital care was provided by local governments. In that year, the first federal domiciliary and medical facility was established—the U.S. Naval Home in Philadelphia.

With America's growth as a nation, and its increasing involvement in armed conflict—War of 1812, Mexican War, Indian Wars, Civil War, Spanish-American War—resulting in greater numbers of maimed and war-injured veterans, Congress by the time of World War I was forced to react in a concerted and uniform way. It did, in 1921, creating the modern beginnings of what ultimately was called the Veterans Administration. By establishing the Veterans Bureau, Congress gathered under one roof the previously disparate responsibilities of the Bureau of War Risk Insurance and those functions of the Public Health Service relating to physical exams and the care and treatment of veterans.

In 1922, to complete its changeover to the functional and administrative predecessor of the present-day VA, the Bureau took charge of the Public Health Service hospitals serving veterans. It is here that the VA legacy becomes intriguing—and enlightening.

One year later, in 1923, Charles Forbes, the first director of the Veterans Bureau, was more humiliated than hurt when he was nearly strangled to death in the White House by his friend, President Warren G. Harding, the man who had personally and enthusiastically selected him in 1921 to head the new, enlarged agency.

Forbes survived the presidential attack only to wind up in Leavenworth federal prison, after a profitable two-year stewardship of the already faltering agency. As a regular poker-playing chum and intimate of Harding—along with, among others, Attorney General Harry Daugherty and Interior Secretary Albert Fall of Teapot Dome fame—the ubiquitous Forbes created a personal and lucrative money machine out of the VA's forerunner. This set the tone for the future Veterans Administration.

Forbes's quarter-billion dollars in accumulated graft, corruption, and inefficiency was to become a landmark by which a succession of VA administrators could be measured.

Forbes warmed up for his Veterans Bureau escapades when, fifteen years after he had been declared a marine deserter, President Woodrow Wilson named him director of construction at

Pearl Harbor. It was in that position that he met President-to-be Warren Harding. (It is, perhaps, a measure of Forbes's political acumen that accounts of his military career differ, particularly with regard to dates and branch of service, or how, despite his early AWOL status, he gained the rank of lieutenant colonel as well as the Congressional Medal of Honor. All agree, however, that he unerringly knew how to sniff out the core of power—and locate himself in close proximity.)

At the time of Forbes's appointment in 1921—warmly applauded by his comrades in the American Legion—the army had assumed the responsibility, through a special architectural staff, for site location and the building of new veterans' hospitals. About twenty were completed when Forbes convinced Harding to place all future veterans' hospital construction under the bureau's—i.e., Forbes's—jurisdiction.

Harding also agreed, at his friend's urging, to remove the responsibility for buying and disposing of veterans' supplies from the quartermaster general's bailiwick and put it in the hands of Forbes. Harding's quickly executed executive order placed control of the four dozen or so government warehouses at Perryville, Maryland—filled to bursting with surplus supplies, equipment, and whatnot—on the not unreceptive shoulders of Lieutenant Colonel Forbes.

Thus Forbes, in about the same amount of time it took him to go AWOL as a young soldier, firmly grasped decision-making power that enabled him to determine where and to whom many millions of dollars of government construction funds would go, how much to charge for huge quantities of allegedly surplus medical and other supplies, and who would help him run the nation's burgeoning number of veterans' services.

He undertook his boldly consolidated mandate with a relish and venality outstanding in the history of U.S. government abuse and scandal—all in the name of the American veteran. The VA, heir to the foundation he laid, is, more than half a century later, still coping with some of the decisions he made.

Francis Russell, in his engaging and controversial biography, *The Shadow of Blooming Grove: Warren G. Harding in His Time,* describes the massive drain from the federal treasury.

As soon as Forbes had taken charge of the Perryville warehouses, he pressured the Bureau of the Budget into giving him blanket approval for the sale of a three-page list of supplies he claimed were damaged. To this list he appended two unapproved lists of his own. Then, with an unconcern that amounted to bravado, he proceeded to empty the warehouses of the supplies and equipment accumulated so lavishly during the war years . . . including such hospital necessities as sheets, blankets, towels, gauze, bandages, drugs, and soap. Alcohol and drugs Forbes found most profitable to divert directly into illegal channels. In addition to the hospital supplies, of which there was then a countrywide shortage, there were on the warehouse premises thousands of trucks and vast quantities of tools. Without any publicity, Forbes arranged for this material, which he represented as surplus and practically useless, to go by private bid to a Boston firm, Thompson & Kelley. Two other firms got wind of the sale and submitted bids, but theirs were discredited.

Day after day, the freight cars moved out of Perryville for Boston with their loads. . . . At one point, new sheets were being brought in at one end of a Perryville warehouse and loaded out the other end as surplus.

All in all, Thompson & Kelley bought between $5 and $7 million worth of government goods for which the firm paid $600,000. Forbes was no less lavish in his purchases than in his sales. The Veterans Bureau bought 70,000 gallons of floor wax and cleaner—enough to last a hundred years [and "polish a dance floor half the size of South Dakota," according to later Congressional testimony] at 98 cents a gallon, although its actual value per gallon was 4 cents.

Whatever percentage Forbes received of the Perryville sales, it was trivial compared to the graft he was able to extract from his control of veterans' hospital construction. Congress had appropriated $17 million— and would later double that figure—for needed new hospitals. To replace the Army's well-managed architectural staff, Forbes set up his own architectural sub-department that, although it cost $100,000 a year to run, was so inept that many of its plans had later to be scrapped. The Public Health and Marine Hospital services had been able to build hospitals at a cost of $2,972 a bed. Forbes' architects raised the cost per bed to $4,957.

At Excelsior Springs, Missouri, Forbes agreed to pay $77,000 for land worth $35,000, then raised the price to $90,000.

Russell also recounts how Forbes used his office to land "no-show" jobs for those in his favor.

In an understatement that somehow has escaped being printed

on official VA stationery, Maj. Gen. John F. Ryan, counsel for the Senate investigating committee that examined the bureau's abuses in 1925, observed later that "the great work of aiding the disabled was prostituted to self-aggrandisement and greed."

Despite the mounting evidence, Harding steadfastly refused to believe reports about Forbes's activities. When summoned to the White House for an explanation, Forbes, without batting an eye, reported to his boss that the supplies he was selling were deteriorating and worthless and, as a good administrator, he was simply getting the best price he could while cutting down on storage expenses. In a grand gesture of proof Forbes, portraying himself as unfairly maligned, presented the relieved president with some samples of the purportedly decaying supplies. The American Legion strongly supported the embattled but slippery Forbes, and vociferously criticized anyone who placed fiscal concerns above the higher calling of care of America's veterans.

Eventually, Harding brought himself to acknowledge the felonious ways of his close buddy. His reaction to the news was rather extraordinary.

Author Russell writes,

The next afternoon a visitor to the White House with an appointment to see the President was directed by mistake to the second floor. As he approached the Red Room, he heard a voice hoarse with anger, and on entering saw Harding throttling a man against the wall as he shouted, "You yellow rat! You double-crossing bastard! If you ever . . ." Whirling about at the visitor's approach, Harding loosed his grip and the released man staggered away, his face blotched and distorted. "I am sorry," Harding said curtly to his visitor. "You have an appointment. Come into the next room."

On leaving the White House, the visitor asked a doorman who it was who had just gone out after he had come in, and the doorman replied, "Colonel Forbes of the Veterans Bureau."

Shortly thereafter, with the details of his misdeeds no longer deniable, Forbes sailed to France on the pretext of exploring the needs of surviving disabled veterans. Soon to follow, after a shakeup at the Veterans Bureau had been announced, were resolutions in the Senate and House calling for an investigation into what the Senate labeled allegations of "waste, extravagance, irregularities, and mismanagement" in the Veterans Bureau.

On February 15, Forbes sent a cable to Harding, tendering his resignation.

Reflecting later on the betrayal of trust by one of his closest companions, Harding confided to William Allen White as the two of them rode a train across the Kansas prairie in June 1923. With Congress up in arms over the Veterans Bureau scandal, White, a fellow midwesterner, newspaperman, and sometime booster of the sinking Harding administration, reports that Harding blurted out, in despair, "I have no trouble with my enemies. I can take care of them. It is my friends. My friends that are giving me my trouble!"

Typical of Harding's problems, the quotation, now part of the idiom in altered form, lost its origins along the way. It is generally and erroneously accepted as a by-product of Teapot Dome—which exploded after Harding's death—rather than a nugget of early VA history.

Forbes stood trial in Chicago, along with a construction firm pal also implicated in the mess, on charges of bribery and conspiracy. On the next to last day of January 1925, two years after resigning from his position, Forbes was found guilty. His penalty for looting some $225,000,000 from the American taxpayers was two years in Leavenworth and a $100,000 fine.

But the scandal's aftermath went farther still.

As if to punctuate the disaster that had befallen the doomed agency, Charles Cramer, a participant in many of Forbes's money-making schemes and not so incidentally also general counsel for the Veterans Bureau, took it upon himself, as the disgrace spread, to place a .45-caliber pistol against his right temple and pull the trigger.

Among Cramer's legacies was his brokering of a payment of $105,000 by the bureau for some land at Livermore, California, which was valued at $19,257 by an official of the state American Legion. Cramer got $12,500 for his troubles; Forbes the same.

Today, the 186-bed Livermore VA Medical Center stands on the site.

With the exit of Forbes, Harding quickly took measures to ensure that not even a taint of corruption would ever again besmirch the fallen standard of the Veterans Bureau. Accordingly, early in 1923 he named as Forbes's successor Brig. Gen. Frank T. Hines, a bald-pated, slightly built, shipbuilding businessman who spent the next twenty-two years trying to keep the Veterans Bureau (and, beginning in 1930, the Veterans Administration) from the pit of financial corruption.

And he did. Unfortunately, in the process Hines established another VA tradition, one just as insidious if not as venal.

It was an era that saw the VA regularly deny much-needed equipment and supplies to its far-flung beleaguered staff in the name of fiscal restraint. Hines's actions even provoked the normally sympathetic American Legion, which, in exasperation, expended some $3,500 of its own monies to provide vital medical materials (radium, in this case) for the men on the wards.

Shortages, lamented the Legion, were the result of "general pressure(s) for economical administration."

In 1945, Albert Deutsch, a muckraking journalist, testified from his articles in *PM* before one of a stream of House (and Senate) investigating committees that were to become as familiar as the VA itself.

"In his efforts to end money dishonesty . . . ," Deutsch wrote, "Hines paved the way for other abuses and defects. He placed excessive stress on paper work. Bureaucratic procedures developed, which tied up the organization in needless red tape. Avoidance of scandal became the main guide of official action. Anything new was discouraged: 'It might get us in trouble.' Routineers and mediocrities rose to high office by the simple process of not disturbing the status quo. Good men were frozen out or quit. . . . the agency increasingly was controlled by old men with old ideas."

Hines and his aides, Deutsch told the Congress members, jealously guarded their bastion from intruding outsiders. "The VA remains the sacred cow of Washington, immune to official investigation, above questioning—almost a dictatorially governed domain within the Federal Government." Deutsch called Hines's attitude toward medicine "medieval," a perspective that discouraged good doctors from entering the VA system and risked the health of patients by delaying the use of new medication, equipment, and procedures.

Hines defended his position, asserting that he refused to let hospitalized veterans be used as "guinea pigs" in "experimentation" with unproven drugs by "inexperienced doctors." Ironically, the very same words are used today—by veterans who object to the use of their bodies as learning labs for the testing of the emerging skills of newly anointed physicians: Hines's bureaucratic chickens coming home to roost.

In addition, Hines, a conservative Republican in a spendthrift New Deal administration, smugly bragged of the regularity with which he returned unexpended monies to the federal coffers, thereby reversing his predecessor's acquisitive habits with a vengeance. By then, as the Second World War was winding down, the VA system, having in 1930 assumed the burden of two more agencies administering veterans' benefits, had already swelled to 53,000 employees potentially serving more than 16 million veterans. Its annual budget was now $1.12 million, supporting ninety-four facilities with 100,000 beds.

The needs, nonetheless, went unmet.

Testified Deutsch,

There was only one social worker at this institution [Northport, New York, VA] accommodating 2,800 patients. At least three more were needed, but the Veterans Administration has been unable to recruit anywhere near enough of these professionals at the low base pay it offers, $2,000 a year.

The total budget for all Veterans Administration psychiatric research amounted to only $25,000 a year, pitiably inadequate. . . . Only 17 psychiatrists had been trained at this center [Northport, the VA's research and training facility] since its establishment 2 years ago. The Army Neuropsychiatric Division had given psychiatric training to more than 200 young doctors in the same period.

Veterans suffered in other ways. Albert Maisel, who wrote a series of VA exposés for *Cosmopolitan,* testified before the same House Committee on World War Veterans' Legislation:

The complaints [at Castle Point, New York, VA] ran in terms of over-charging [at the canteen], but particularly—they also alleged that the man was also running a horse-betting parlor and similar things, but the particular complaint was that he operated this canteen which prepared food which the patients ate . . . that this canteen prepared food without the use of a sterilizer in washing the dishes, and that therefore positive sputum from TB cases, contagious cases, were using dishes which were then passed on with just a rinse or wash to the patients, to nontubercular patients, and to the negative sputum cases.

The House committee heard from the Veterans of Foreign Wars, too. Frank M. Whitaker, the VFW department service officer for New York, reported that the shortage of ward attend-ants "is not only serious, but is very dangerous, particularly in the violent wards." In one ward, he noted, "Forty-eight violent pa-tients are in charge of [*sic*] two attendants."

Whitaker, testifying about numerous beatings and frequent physical violence at VA hospitals from coast to coast, goes on, "The enlisted men assigned by the Army, particularly, are not qualified to act as hospital attendants and might well be classified as Army 'misfits.' We were informed they were assigned these hospital duties when it was decided they were not adaptable to other military duties."

As the head of a fact-finding group, he concludes, "The com-mittee is of the opinion that the Veterans Administration at cen-tral office [in Washington, D.C.] is out of complete touch with the situation and has no realization of the condition and needs of the Northport facility."

Maisel, whose 1945 article "Third-Rate Medicine for First-Rate Men" caused a national uproar, suggests his experiences were the same, but his examples are subtler.

"Our tour took us into another crowded dayroom," Maisel re-calls. "Dr. Hoffman noticed a patient wearing the cuffs. 'Do those restraints hurt?' he asked the man.

" 'No,' came the slow response. The veteran stared at his hands awhile. Finally he added, 'These things don't hurt me here.' He lifted his shackled right hand as far as the belt would let it go, and tried to point it toward his heart. 'It's here where they hurt,' he said."

The twenty members of the House Committee on World War Veterans' Legislation listened to more than thirty-three days of often impassioned testimony over a period of eight months. (The official transcript exceeded 2,600 pages in seven volumes.)

But the bottom line came up fuzzy.

Eight of the twenty members issued a minority report which asserted that the VA "was not equipped to provide the best quality of modern medicine." They pointed to an overabundance of "complacency and inflexibility in some of the administrative heads." They recommended expansion of VA contact with the outside medical community, an upgrading of physicians, nurses, and other staff, increased installation of modern equipment in hospitals, and the creation of additional research opportunities.

The majority, for its part, satisfied with the appointment of a new administrator (Hines had "resigned" before the hearings ended) and aggravated by the uppitiness of some of the witnesses, drew a collective sigh of relief and graciously let bygones be bygones. The brief report concluded that "conditions in veterans' hospitals were neither as bad as portrayed by the periodicals or individuals, nor were they everything desired by this committee."

Satisfied that what they thought was a small amount of patient abuse was being properly dealt with (several VA personnel were indicted) and pleased with a new law, Public Law 293, which created a Department of Medicine and Surgery in the VA, the majority of the committee proceeded to wash its hands clean of the entire affair.

Benjamin Lewis, a longtime employee in the VA's Department of Medicine and Surgery, gingerly writes, "It is safe to conclude that veterans' medicine up to World War II was practiced under conditions which would not assure a continuing diffusion of the highest standards of medical care throughout the system." Even the VA itself got into the act. In a public statement, it called its own professional staff levels "far below adequate and desirable."

"The Veterans Administration hospitals are in the backwaters of American medicine," a prominent physician stated flatly, "where doctors stagnate and where patients who deserve the best must often be satisfied with second-rate treatment."

Enter General Omar N. Bradley.

Bradley, the "GI's general," served as VA administrator for only two years, 1945–47, the shortest tenure of all except for Forbes. It was a time of genuine promise and accomplishment in an agency where leadership and sensitivity, not to mention honesty and compassion, were sorely lacking.

Under Bradley, whom many observers consider the only capable administrator the VA has ever seen, the agency spewed out benefits efficiently, with unprecedented consistency: VA hospitals were handling 85 percent more patients in only 44 percent more beds; in some hospitals, the average length of stay per patient was cut by as much as two-thirds; the GI Bill, said to have had more impact on the American way of life than any law since the passage of the Homestead Act more than a century ago, saw millions of returning soldiers take advantage of educational and training programs; home loans under the bill soared; the appointment of VA physicians, dentists, and nurses was removed from the stultifying limitations of the Civil Service statutes; and clinical psychology was recognized as a helping profession.

Complaints about the treatment afforded veterans virtually disappeared.

The most far-reaching decision during Bradley's stay was the enactment of Public Law 293, signed on January 3, 1946, by President Truman, which established the Department of Medicine and Surgery. Now the VA, in the running of its medical program at least, was free of Civil Service restraints. It quickly set about to hire the best medical professionals in the country, and that meant going to the medical schools.

Bradley, the disciplined administrator and master of the chain of command, chose his top aides wisely. Foremost among them were his former chief surgeon in Europe, Maj. Gen. Paul R. Hawley, whom he named to head the new department, and Dr. Paul

Magnuson, a farsighted and self-confident surgeon, as Hawley's deputy. The two men transformed the agency.

With Bradley's encouragement and approval, they immediately set out to forge the Forbes-Hines legacy of an abusive system into a model of modern health care. Eagerly and aggressively, the pair traveled around the country, suggesting the removal of unsatisfactory personnel from individual hospitals while wooing department chairmen of medical schools into the heretofore chilling embrace of the VA.

The major vehicle for this latter effort was their famous Policy Memorandum No. 2, a directive issued January 30, 1946, that forever altered the mandate of the VA. With no specific legal authorization, Hawley and Magnuson committed the VA's vast medical complex to a sharing of its facilities and staff with medical schools throughout the country.

Through a mechanism called the Deans' Committee, the memorandum outlines the two parties' responsibilities: The VA will retain full responsibility for the care of patients, including professional treatment, and the school of medicine accepts responsibility for all graduate education and training. The Deans' Committee, composed of senior faculty members of the medical school, nominates the consultants, part-time attending staff, and the residents; the VA does the approving.

In short, for the first time in anyone's memory, a federal agency gave up some of its hiring and administrative prerogatives to an outside, nongovernment entity. Training of doctors now became part of the VA package, which until then contained only the treatment and care of eligible veterans. When it worked well, it worked very well. When it didn't—well, the ghosts of Forbes and Hines were invoked.

"Those were exciting days in the Veterans Administration Medical Department," Magnuson, as virulently antibureaucratic as one can be, recalls in his self-congratulatory autobiography, *Ring the Night Bell.* He recounts his efforts to convince several northern California medical schools to come aboard.

"You've got a [VA] hospital here which is easily accessible to both of your medical schools and you can set up your own teaching program and *appoint your own staff,"* he told one such meeting. "Now when do we go to work?" (Italics added.) When the dean of the University of California Medical School, after a moment's pause, says, "How about eight o'clock tomorrow morning?" Magnuson is elated.

He is equally delighted when, after telling the deans of Tufts, Boston University, and Harvard medical schools that the VA would build a hospital anywhere they wanted it and "thereafter it would be *up to them to staff it,"* they agreed to do it. (Italics added.)

These promises, as stated by Magnuson, directly violated the letter, not to say the spirit, of Policy Memorandum No. 2. In his enthusiasm, Dr. Magnuson had put down the groundwork for some terrible problems to come. In fact, a warning, sounded early, was duly noted, and then ignored.

Cautions a Special Committee of the Subcommittee on Hospitals of the House Committee on Veterans Affairs, June 19, 1947.

The Veterans Administration should be held responsible for the treatment of the veterans and patients and they should see to it that the hospital does not become a training ground for medical students rather than a veterans' hospital with the veterans' receiving proper treatment. The Veterans Administration should also be careful that the control of the veterans' hospital is not lost to the staff of the medical schools that are being used to instruct the resident doctors.

The report was to prove prophetic.

Very few objected to the growing connections between hospitals and the schools, glowingly portrayed earlier by such authorities as those participating in a 1923 hospital consultants survey for the Treasury Department who stated, even then, that "the very best type of medical care given is in those institutions that come under the critical eye of students and in which teaching is carried out."

Rather, the concern turned to the use of veterans as captive subjects forced to submit to inexperienced, perhaps insensitive, trainees sent to VA hospitals by a school more interested in what its students could get out of the experience than in the health of the patients. The Veterans of Foreign Wars, though no longer vociferously critical of the practice, adopted a resolution as late as 1962 condemning the medical schools for "giving more attention to the training program than to the welfare of the patients," resulting, it added, in "inadequate and sometimes inexperienced medical attention."

Like the trail of corruption and insensitive, irrational bureaucratic frugality blazed by his two predecessors, Bradley's small bend in the road, while noted for its noble purposes and implementation of clear-eyed, progressive policies, nonetheless added to the spoors along the wayside.

How quickly things reverted to their previous state—and a measure of the government's resurgent attitude toward its used-up war heroes—can be seen in the choice of Bradley's successor.

As were all the administrators before him, Carl R. Gray, Jr., was a high-ranking military officer. A major general during the war, and in 1947 vice-president of the Chicago and Northwestern Railroad, Gray wasted no time in alienating the very people who had revitalized the burgeoning agency. He was a bureaucrat's bureaucrat.

Soon after he joined the VA, Gray developed a blockage of the central vision in one eye. He had already acquired an almost complete deficit of vision in the other eye, so that he was unable to read typewritten words.

"Once in a while I saw him get out a big magnifying glass and try to decipher a letter on his desk, but I never saw him finish one," writes Magnuson, who finally was fired after a bitter battle with the doltish Gray. "So, the only letters he ever knew about were the ones his staff chose to read to him. He couldn't study a chart in detail, he couldn't get any information except what the bureaucrats who swarmed in his office told him."

One of the things Gray, who stayed five years, did with his time —and poor eyesight—was to tour all the VA hospitals. The trip, which took all of nine months and pretty much kept him away from his desk in Washington, still stands as a monument to the now frizzled conceit implicit in the VA's public relations homily that it extends to the American veteran medical care second to none.

Magnuson reports:

He would start at one end of a corridor and march vigorously down it, ducking in every door on the right side to give a quick and seemingly penetrating glance at what was going on inside the room or ward. Then he turned around at the end of the corridor and did the same thing at each door on the left side, and continued this until he had been in every room in the hospital.

People found this performance impressive unless they knew the truth, which was that he was not seeing one single thing he was looking at, and if he had been able to see it, it would not have meant anything to him, because he knew nothing about hospitals.

For reasons undocumented, Gray was the last veterans' affairs administrator who came along with a military title. But he wasn't the last military-involved administrator. The VA, looking for leadership (and the presidents who did the appointing looking for votes), traded in the uniform for a legionnaire's cap.

Five of the last six VA administrators (last seven if former President Carter's appointee, Max Cleland, is counted) have held high positions in a veterans' service organization. Included are two former national commanders of the American Legion and one commander in chief of the Veterans of Foreign Wars. There is also an ex-Massachusetts lieutenant governor and a former Georgia legislator who tried to be a lieutenant governor.

The move in this direction was based on several factors, but its goal was singular—to defuse the increasingly strident criticism that was coming mainly from relatively unorganized veterans as well as nonveterans' groups—and, occasionally, from some quarters of Congress. The same kind of public relations thinking was involved in President Carter's calculated choice of Cleland, a personable triple-amputee Vietnam veteran, as administrator when criticism of the VA by younger veterans was beginning to boil.

Traditionally, the various service organizations tended to steer away from any sort of in-depth, detailed faultfinding of a system that by and large treated them well. Early on, the VA made certain it would keep a long tether attached when it gave free office space in VA facilities to representatives of the major veterans' service groups. Members of these organizations are frequently close personal friends of VA administrators (or are themselves VA administrators) and generally limit their energies to lobbying for more and increased bonuses and pension benefits. Concern about the quality of medical care and hospitalization, on the other hand, has not been abundant, for two reasons.

One, the bigwigs in the service organizations get markedly better care than the ordinary veteran. Codes on their medical charts, identifying their status, alert the staff to treat them accordingly. (Sometimes the preferred treatment starts at the door. At least one hospital, Philadelphia, has accepted telephone calls in advance from visiting service officers for reserved parking space in the VA lot, thereby eliminating the hassle of fighting for the rare legal street spot in the crowded downtown area.)

And secondly, the bulk of the organizations' membership, generally well established in their communities, does not make regular use of the VA when their paid-up medical insurance can get them into the private hospitals of their choice. The typical user —elderly, no longer able to earn a living because of the cumulative effects of age and war disabilities, refused medical insurance for those very reasons—presents a profile different from that of the successful Legionnaire or VFW post commander.

"There is a class difference between the service organization as provider and the veterans as users," says Columbia University's Michael Sklar.

But circumstances may be altering that reality. Since VA patients are increasingly older and less able to pay for their own health care, and since the World War II veteran, who makes up the vast majority of the major service organizations, is himself increasingly older and sicker, the American Legion and other similar groups are beginning to show signs of exerting more pressure on the VA to upgrade facilities that more and more of their members will be using in the future.

And they can apply that pressure, too, as they have over the years. For example, up until ten years or so ago, any annual budget request to Congress by the VA was in effect automatically *increased* by the appropriate Senate and House committees. Generally, these increases affected compensation and pension benefits, rather than medical care, and often they were passed at the urging of the service organizations.

Over the years, the veterans' groups have also successfully lobbied for the inclusion of additional war-related injuries and diseases on the compensation lists. But hard financial times no longer allow for swollen budgets, and shifting alliances have weakened somewhat the power balance in the incestuous relationships among the three components of the so-called iron triangle—the VA, the veterans' affairs committees in Congress, and the service organizations themselves.

For example, Ralph Casteel, a VA employee for thirty-three years, including long stints as an assistant to more than one chief medical director, is currently a staff member of the House Committee on Veterans' Affairs, specializing in legislative and oversight matters. He is openly antagonistic toward his former associates.

Oliver Meadows, now retired, was for twenty-five years staff director for the House Committee before being elected national commander of the Disabled American Veterans in 1977. And Richard Roudebush, Cleland's immediate predecessor, managed to touch all three bases before retiring: VFW national commander; member, as an elected representative, of the Veterans' Affairs Committee; and, after failing in a bid for the Senate, special assistant to then-VA administrator Donald Johnson, himself a former national commander of the American Legion.

"This sort of internal cohesiveness no doubt fosters the best of relations among those concerned with setting policy," writes Paul Starr in *The Discarded Army: Veterans After Vietnam.* "But it also raises questions about the potential for feedback and adaptation." That is, who's watching the henhouse?

An embarrassing example of this mutual back-scratching arrangement surfaced during the 1945 Hines hearings. For most of the sessions, the American Legion, the VFW, and DAV sat quietly and listened. Less than a week after Hines's forced resignation, the service groups, realizing a new, independent administrator was about to come aboard, quickly jumped on the bandwagon. Their belated, but critical, statements before the investigating committee made front-page headlines from New York to California.

At about the time of those hearings, an experienced VA physician complained,

Blame can be spread everywhere, but many of us feel that the veterans' organizations are largely at fault. In my seven years' service with the VA, I have often heard the veterans' organizations clamor for more monetary benefits and I have seen them maneuver for special privileges, but I never saw them exert themselves to raise the VA's standards of medical treatment. How come . . . ?

The service organizations acquire their power from large memberships; they recruit large memberships through offers of greater monetary benefits and special privileges. . . .

Now what has this to do with the standards of medical treatment in the VA? Mainly this: Veterans' organizations have most use for docile physicians and executives. Such men have been rewarded with the leading positions in many but not all instances. Many good men have resigned in disgust.

The VFW proudly disseminated two years ago a well-designed glossy pamphlet extolling its eighty-year record of achievement. Of the sixty-eight achievements listed, only eight directly concern themselves with hospital-medical care. More than one-third deal with pensions and similar cash benefits. One tells of the VFW's long history of recommending legislation to outlaw the U.S. Communist party.

But as a younger generation came home from war—a generation not uncomfortable with voicing its demands for its rights and benefits—the complexion of the cozy relationship, and, hence, the iron triangle's mission, began to change. The young vets, by not joining the service organizations in the droves they once did after earlier, less complicated wars, accomplished two things. First, they drained away some of the clout from an already declining membership. Secondly, the service groups, desperate for new members, began slowly to express some sympathy toward the younger vets' complaints and needs.

This was especially true of the DAV. As a result, it has blossomed into a broad-based outfit, leading the way (even over the VA) in programs specifically and carefully designed for the returned young veteran. Today, the DAV boasts a growing membership, of which some 25 percent are Vietnam veterans. With constituencies concerned about medical care (and other critical benefits, such as job training) the service organizations are now rethinking their involvement in those areas.

Even the VA has felt the effect.

Partially by virtue of the success of the DAV's Forgotten Warrior project, Congress finally followed suit, forking over $10 million in 1979 to the VA for its own counseling outreach program. Cleland calls the outreach programs, based in a community storefront rather than in the usual government building, innovative and new. It might be new to the VA, but places like Lincoln Hospital/Albert Einstein College of Medicine in the South Bronx and community mental health centers in Boston, Chicago, and elsewhere pioneered the concept at about the time Cleland was accepting the Atlanta *Journal* trophy as the outstanding senior in his Lithonia High School graduating class, some two decades ago.

Almost in self-defense, then, Presidents Eisenhower, Kennedy, Johnson, Nixon, and Ford—cognizant of the organizations' don't-rock-the-boat history and responsive to political realities—made sure that every appointee in the fifties, sixties, and early to mid-seventies was a former top service officer; the one exception, LBJ's 1965 pick of William J. Driver, was a World War II–Korean War veteran who became the first (and, so far, last) career official to administer the affairs of America's veterans.

The choice of representatives from organized, highly visible veterans' groups serves another, more generalized, purpose as well. By mixing the military with civilian programs, the government-veterans' alliance maintains a public climate that unobtrusively but consistently includes a familiar, benign military presence even in peacetime. As a result, it makes for smoother recruiting when the public relations drums are periodically beaten to let the citizenry—including potential soldiers and veterans—know what might await them when and if they return from battle.

The VA, Paul Starr correctly points out, "is a cross between the Pentagon and [the former] HEW. . . . The VA is that point in the federal government where the demands for guns and butter resonate. . . . Benefits also facilitate social control within the army. By threatening soldiers with less than honorable discharges, the military can deny them subsequent advantages. Perhaps most important, an extensive system of veterans' services fosters a continued identification with the military among large segments of the population. This strengthens the military's domestic political position."

Sometimes there are problems, and it doesn't matter if a four-star general, a combined American Legion–VFW commander, or the entire U.S. Congress is at the helm.

By mid-1970, with the ferocity of the Vietnam War unrelenting, some 275,000 Americans were counted as wounded. Chances of surviving a battle injury in Vietnam were much better than those for World War II and Korea. Eighty-one percent of army troops wounded in Vietnam survived compared with 71 percent in the Second World War. Quick attention on the battlefield, highly efficient helicopter evacuation, and sophisticated medical advances ensured a higher number of lives saved—and incredible overcrowding in stateside VA hospitals.

VA statistics showed at the time, for example, that paraplegia (loss of use of the lower part of the body) had an incidence close to 1,000 percent higher than that incurred in combat twenty-five years earlier. Men were surviving, but they weren't necessarily getting healthy any more quickly. One result, VA data also revealed, was that of those wounded in Vietnam, one out of seven would wind up in what *Life* in a cover-story exposé that year called "the bleak backwaters of our Veterans Administration hospitals."

Bobby Muller, a paraplegic paralyzed from the chest down, turned out to be one of those one in seven. And, in the train of a

VA history which saw the likes of Colonel Forbes at the newly welded controls, the Kingsbridge VA Medical Center in the Bronx turned out to be one of the VA's "bleak backwaters." The two came together ten years ago, and the experience for both of them, born of fifty-plus years of VA health care second to none, was not pleasant. It is the VA's biography. And lurking in the shadows is a full cast of characters—from Forbes to Cleland.

Muller, now a vigorous advocate of the rights of Vietnam (and all) veterans, was a young marine lieutenant leading a South Vietnamese unit up a heat-choked hill near the refugee village of Cam Lo. It was the twilight of an April evening in 1969, and the jet fighters and artillery called in by Lieutenant Muller seemed to have no effect on the machine guns manned by the North Vietnamese, who wanted the battered real estate as much as the Americans and their allies did.

The gunfire was intense and unrelenting. Suddenly, the sky, ebbing into nighttime, seemed to cave in. Muller, at the head of the assault, caught a bullet through his chest and both lungs.

He was slammed to the ground, his spinal cord severed. He would never walk again. Lying on the bloodstained battlefield, he thought he would never breathe again.

Less than two months later, Muller, from Queens, New York, was wheeled into the Kingsbridge VA hospital, a dirty, turn-of-the-century amalgam of antiquated red-brick buildings on land once part of the Ringling Brothers circus (later an orphanage), and leftover World War II Quonset huts. Overcrowded and reeking of nauseating smells, sunlight barely pierced the gloom of the dank hallways.

"It was a filthy, dirty place," remembers a technologist who worked for a short time in 1974 in the hospital's bacteriology lab. "It was so sad, such a depressing place. We found a mouse in a drawer which had sterile pipettes. This mouse jumped out. I mentioned it to another person and he opened another drawer, one with sterile tissue grinders. The drawer had mouse droppings in it." Muller recalls that the mere sight of the place brought him to tears. The treatment, he found out quickly enough, equaled the physical conditions. It transformed him.

"The day I got to the hospital, I asked for a wheelchair. They said, 'No, we can't get you one. We don't have any.' I went crazy. I said, 'Get me a goddamn wheelchair,' started screaming, pissing, and moaning, and this wasn't me. I want you to know that. This is very important. I had been a marine. If I had a superior, it was 'Yes, sir. No, sir.' It wasn't my nature to yell back at doctors. It wasn't my nature to go to authority figures and those in charge and, you know, go against them. But, goddamn it, when you're backed into a corner and it's a matter of your personal survival, I don't care who it is, you're going to either sink or come out fighting, and that's what I had to do: get me the wheelchair."

Muller stops talking for a moment. He looks gaunt against the darkening sky outside his cluttered office on the ninth floor of a nondescript building on Park Avenue South in New York City, headquarters for his Vietnam Veterans of America.

It is hard to talk about a medical slum, where even, as in a real slum, the basic, everyday necessities are absent.

Ron Kovic, a two-tour marine who shared some of the misery with Muller at Kingsbridge, describes, in his autobiography, *Born on the Fourth of July*, what he was told when he learned the hospital didn't have certain life-supporting equipment he desperately needed. All they could offer him was worn-out, faltering machinery.

"The young doctor explains in a very matter-of-fact way that this is the only pump they have," Kovic, also paraplegic, writes. "It all has to do with the war, he explains. It is all because of the war. 'The government is not giving us money for things that we need.' "

Muller straightens up in his wheelchair, remembering.

"Dr. S. I'll never forget him. He was the chief of the department. He came by, I think, the second or third day I was in the hospital, and he said, 'Well, Muller, you've got a transected spinal cord. You know that means you're never going to walk again, don't you?'

"I said, 'Doctor, is there a complete severance there?' I said this to him in this incredulous manner. He said, 'Yes, yes. You've really got to settle with this fact.' And in ten seconds he was gone.

"I was stunned, and I sat there with my mouth open and I told the woman behind the doctor—she was a psychologist—I said, 'I got to see you, I got to talk with you. I don't believe this guy. I've got to talk to somebody.'

"I had just come from the naval hospital at St. Albans and had spoken at great length with the top neurologist and he told me, because I was so critical at the time, it was a real photo finish for me, that they never did anything on the back. They never opened it up. They never did a laminectomy to take a look at the spinal cord. He said nobody can tell with any certainty what the extent of the damage really was. 'We can try to approximate [your status] with the x-rays and the bone fragments, but we don't know for sure.'

"The whole point is, with the spinal cord it's very hard to make any sort of a definitive statement. And here is this jerk, the chief, who gets to meet me as he's coming up to my bed with a three-by-five card that has some rough notes, and he makes an absolute statement without any qualifiers, that, yes, that's it, you've got a complete transection of the cord, there's absolutely no chance that any improvement will be realized.

"And I was stunned, because I knew that prudence in the profession requires that you don't make off-the-cuff remarks in such an absolute manner. This guy was to me, in the professional sense, an imbecile. And he's the top doctor here? Holy Christ.

"Then, literally two weeks later, the same guy came on grand rounds again. I said I wanted braces, and he said, 'You can't have braces.'

"I said, 'Why?'

"He said, 'You have too high a level of injury. You'll never ambulate.'

"And I was stunned again because I had been going to therapy over the past week and they said they'll try and get me on braces and ambulate.

"The following Monday, I had my consultation with an outside physician, Dr. Abrahamson, who was a surgeon in the Second World War and bought a piece of shrapnel in his back. Became a paraplegic. Abrahamson came in and asked how I was doing. I said, 'Terrible, doctor.'

"He said, 'What's the matter?'

"I said, 'They didn't get me braces here.'

"Now, Abrahamson is a paraplegic himself who wears his braces every day.

"He said, 'Who wouldn't give you braces?'

"I said, 'The chief of the department!'

"Now, everybody was there—the nurses, the aides, the therapists, the doctors, and this guy tore Dr. S. a new asshole, right in front of me.

"Abrahamson said, 'Don't you ever deny a paraplegic the right to have braces so that he can try and ambulate. Whether he does or not is irrelevant. The fact is that he wants to try, and you should not come in and take away that right and that option he has to at least attempt to make it happen.'

"I felt much better. I got my braces, of course, as did every other veteran who ever came through that hospital after that."

Dr. Arthur Abrahamson, head of the rehabilitation service at Kingsbridge from 1950–55 (and still a consultant) and since then chairman of the Department of Rehabilitation Medicine at Albert Einstein College of Medicine, says, "I would say what happened to Muller was more widespread than need be—it still is. You gotta be sharp there. They're not sharp there."

Robert O. Muller is sharp. He is also an animated, forceful speaker, thinner than he looks in his marine photos, and intense. Handicapped or not, he jets from one end of the country to the other, gathering support for his Vietnam Veterans of America (VVA), the first national organization dealing solely with the needs, rights, and problems of Vietnam veterans.

VVA is one of those groups—Swords-to-Plowshares, Flower of the Dragon, National Association of Concerned Veterans (NACV), the Center for Veterans' Rights are some others—which has grown out of the war's aftermath and the general coolness displayed toward the younger vets by the traditional service organizations—and by the VA. Muller's group is the largest, with the possible exception of NACV, and he is determined to turn it into a powerful national lobbying and educational force.

A law school graduate and magnificent orator whose organizational skills earlier found expression in involvement with Viet-

nam Veterans Against the War and as legislative director for the
Eastern Paralyzed Veterans Association, Muller is not afraid to
take on Max Cleland on his own turf. Both men are in their late
thirties, war-injured, and dependent on a wheelchair to get
around. The similarity ends there: Muller, the aggressive, articulate, bright, committed protagonist; Cleland, the moderating,
careful, honey-voiced, whirlwind, all-American political appointee. Justice, some say, would surely have placed Muller in Cleland's VA wheelchair.

"It's no contest," says someone who knows them both.

It has grown dark outside the VVA offices, almost dark as night,
even though it isn't yet 5 P.M. on a late August workday. Thunder
and lightning accompany an enormous rainstorm. Muller, tired
from the day and the prospect of several more hours of complicated, tedious organizational planning still ahead, is wound up, a
not uncommon manifestation when he is arguing the case for the
Vietnam veteran, or against an insensitive, abusive bureaucracy.

His forcefulness cuts through the dusk. He continues:

"At the VA, we had one set of parallel bars with, sometimes,
twenty-five guys in wheelchairs waiting for an opportunity to get
between the parallel bars and do these stretching exercises. We
had two therapists. I spent most of that year waiting for my turn.
When we petitioned the administrator of the hospital, he said, 'We
don't have any money, we don't have any appropriations. We're
out of money.' " Muller's anger is racing now, pouring forth in a
hot and disciplined stream from the boy who once refused to
criticize his elders, now a man intent on establishing just where
the responsibility lies. "No money?" he repeats, astounded at the
evil of the words.

"This, mind you, was a rap they gave to me, a guy who was a
marine infantry officer who, literally on occasion, had the battle-
ship *New Jersey* in support of me, who on many occasions called
in, literally, not figuratively, hundreds of thousands of dollars of
supportive arms in jet strikes, artillery, continuous barrages, to
fucking kill people, and now you're telling me after I got shot in
the process that it's all of a sudden inflationary, 'fiscally irresponsible,' to quote Richard Nixon, to try and provide us anything that
resembles adequate care.

"Bullshit. I said, your priorities are crazy and most people who heard that statement would agree with it."

But the obstacles went further, were, in a sense, subtler.

"Then we had all the foreign doctors. I had fucking nightmares from the goddamn system with all the Oriental doctors. Now, mind you, one thing that I try very, very hard to be is sensitive to racism and a host of things like that. Goddamn it, I sure didn't need a bunch of Korean and Oriental doctors being my doctors after having gotten fucking blown away, you know. And it bothered me, and I'll be candid about it."

On May 22, 1970, *Life* magazine published a photo essay. Some of Bobby Muller's and Ron Kovic's friends were in the story, which documented the squalor of the Kingsbridge VA, its rats and garbage on the wards, its shortage of staff, its publicly accessible operating areas, the anguish and despair of its patients. *Life* quotes a lance corporal: "Nobody should have to live in these conditions. We're all hooked up to urine bags, and without enough attendants to empty them, they spill over the floor. It smells and cakes something awful. . . . It's like you've been put in jail, or you've been punished for something."

The rats were the worst part, the lance corporal, a quadriplegic, adds.

But none of that—the photos of signs warning of a leaky roof over a bed, of piles of dirty linen, of seething bitterness—none of it would have made the media splash it did without some outside help. It's a story that has not been told before, something Bobby Muller most likely didn't know back then, perhaps even a little sidelight unknown to many VA officials themselves.

When *Life* came poking through the wards, recording with cameras and notepads the nether regions of a medical slum, indeed, a national disgrace, it was guided not by pure journalistic instincts but by a very knowledgeable aide to some very powerful Congress members. It is a tale that pits two sides of the iron triangle against the third.

The *Life* exposé "was totally contrived. We helped them all the way," asserts Oliver Meadows, the now retired past national commander of the Disabled American Veterans and former staff director for the House Veterans' Affairs Committee, a congressional compendium so synonymous with veterans and VA legislation and oversight that its former long-term chairman, Rep. Olin "Tiger" Teague, has a new VA hospital named for him in his hometown of Temple, Texas. Other congressional VA friends have had similar monuments established through the years.

According to Meadows, the nation's media were constantly being fed so much pap from the VA public relations machine— then-administrator Donald Johnson was trumpeting the canard that veterans could not get better care anywhere in the country— that Meadows and his colleagues on the committee thought nothing short of massive exposure would convince Congress and others otherwise. It also was a matter of muscle flexing, with the veterans' organizations and the committee members determined to assert their authority over an agency that had just rid itself of a non-service organization officer—Driver—who was a career VA official—clearly not one of the good ol' boys.

Meadows, in his role of House committee staff director, coordinated a nationwide information campaign, complete with canned stories and documented lists of assorted hospital horrors. Kingsbridge was just one of many. "The situation was bad, really bad. We went to a lot of trouble to document the problems—places getting dirtier, things not working right. We knew it was the only way to get more money, and break the trend. I did it on my own, with the approval of the chairman [Teague]."

Collecting data from questionnaires sent to the directors of the VA's 166 hospitals, Meadows went to work. "The question we got the most responses to was 'Name the three most pressing problems at your station [hospital].'" He chuckles at the thought.

"We enlisted the aid of the media. We got everybody. We literally staged specials with ABC, NBC, CBS. We staged the network spectaculars. We had major articles in *Reader's Digest, Life* magazine. They were all over the country. We had a specially tailored story written for St. Louis, for example, and the local papers would pick it up. Every VA hospital in the country was covered. We released material to those papers where the hospital was located."

Some VA officials and at least one veteran interviewed for the

Life story claim the stage managing went beyond merely alerting newspapers to allegedly poor conditions at various facilities. They insist that situations at individual hospitals were, in fact, altered and rearranged to create scenes for the cameras that were more sensational than the reality.

Meadows scoffs at those assertions. "We didn't have to arrange things," he says. "Things were bad enough the way they were."

Furthermore, Meadows says he had the explicit support of the committee members. "Of course they knew about it. I was just the producer. The point at the moment was that OMB [Office of Management and Budget] was curtailing the VA budget; it was about to go down the drain. For example, the patient-staff ratio was low. The media simply had to have that kind of background. It was fairly successful. They dug up a half-billion dollars over and above what OMB wanted to give. It was enough to hold body and soul together."

Meadows currently serves on the DAV Committee on Health Services Research, which, says the DAV, is part of "our battle to rescue the VA medical system from the siege being carried out by White House budget cutters." He is eager to do combat with the bureaucrats in the Veterans Administration, and still delights in retelling of his efforts a decade ago to spread the truth about the VA hospital system.

Ten years later, the Kingsbridge hospital hasn't changed much physically. There's more traffic bumping along Kingsbridge Road east to the Grand Concourse and west to the Major Deegan Expressway. True, a brand-new facility has been built, but construction mistakes have delayed its scheduled 1978 opening.

In the outside vestibule entrance to the main building, old yellow newspapers and unidentifiable odors swirl around in the humid wind. Fresh drops of blood line the sidewalk toward the entranceway. At the pharmacy, just inside from the vestibule, some half-dozen people are waiting for their medication. Above the pharmacy windows is a call-board with two rows of brightly colored lights, like a Broadway marquee. The top row is red and displays the numbers of service-connected veterans when their prescription is ready. Underneath, the row of green bulbs iden-

tifies the numbers of non-service-connected vets. The former take
precedence over the latter, making for some spirited discussion
among those who have waited several hours for a single vial of
pills.

Upstairs, on the spinal-cord-injury unit that still causes Muller
to shudder when he thinks about it, the hallway walls are now
painted bright colors and the rooms look clean and well kept. All
five of the men with whom he shared a room are now dead.

"I'm in touch with a lot of guys from the hospital," he says
softly. "My closest friend, my very closest friend, killed himself.
Just out of frustration and disgust. He took every pill in the fucking book. He wrote a note. He had been out of the hospital for a
couple of years, and he said 'later' for this bullshit. So all of that
was what gave the genesis to this fight against the fucking system.
It's not just one hospital. It's the whole system from beginning to
end."

Muller, with the thunder blasting the building outside, is running with his anger again.

"You either survive or you do what most of the guys do, which
is take your compensation check, which is ridiculously high. It's
fucking blood money! They give you more than two thousand
bucks a month, which is what they give me, cold cash, tax-free.
Fine. Sounds great—to anyone who hasn't been shot up. What are
you going to complain about? You've got the equivalent of thirty,
thirty-five thousand dollars' income. The American dream with
a little blood on it.

"You're talking of kids who had an earning expectation of
being a fucking grease mechanic. To them, an eight-thousand-
dollar job would have been a home run. So now you give them the
equivalent of thirty-five thousand, you give them a housing benefit, an adaptive equipment benefit for the automobile.

"Hey, they'll drive their Cadillacs and Eldorados while they're
killing themselves. They have no purpose in life, no fucking
meaning, no sense of self-worth or self-respect. Now they've been
bought off.

"What's the VA done in fifty years? They still don't have meaningful programs. Rather than looking for these guys and giving
them perhaps five business opportunities and setting them up, as

they would in Europe, say, with a kiosk in a very key intersection to do something so they would have a sense of self-worth—no."

Suddenly, a monstrous crack of thunder rattles the office windows. Muller's words are lost in the sky-splitting barrage.

"Here's your fucking money. Go home, kid. That's what they do. They go home and they live with Mom and they're miserable. They watch soap operas all day, becoming fatter," Bobby Muller says as the thunder fades away, "waiting to die."

You go overseas to make provisions for America to stand on its own, then you come back and she stands on you.
—*Black army veteran*

The VA is like a sleeping giant—people don't realize how much it does for the veteran.
—*VA hospital director*

3

AT WAR WITH THE DOCTORS

"No one," says Steve Cannizzaro, "can make a knee like God can."

But the VA, operating under different constraints, can take one away. Or, as Steve's wife Ruby puts it, "This isn't a normal life, not knowing what's going to happen—all the anxiety, all the pressure. It's been very difficult."

Steve Cannizzaro, an army corporal who spent most of his three military service years on the waters of the South Pacific during the early 1940s, is suing the VA for malpractice. And it has nothing to do with his initial encounter with the agency, which came only a few months after an accident resulted in the amputation of his left leg.

Almost immediately, Cannizzaro, fifty-four and a member of the newly created harbor craft unit in World War II, ran into problems at the Long Beach VA. His doctor, a Japanese physician, asked Cannizzaro why he was in the hospital. "He said, 'You veterans. You think you should get everything free,'" Cannizzaro remembers. Upset by the encounter, Cannizzaro didn't return to the VA for five years, preferring instead a private physician in his Indiana hometown. "Although I really couldn't afford it, it was worth the money. At least I wasn't getting insulted," Cannizzaro says. During the five years they were away, Steve developed diabetes. More important for what was to come, however, was the fact that he had been living a normal life with a privately fitted artificial limb, holding down a job, visiting the doctor regularly once a month, and, during icy weather, using a cane.

"I felt that he was able to overcome his handicap in a most excellent manner," wrote the mayor of Montpelier, Indiana, on January 3, 1979, when the ability of Cannizzaro to ambulate had become an issue. "He always walked."

Steve couldn't have been happier with his own progress. "I had no problems whatsoever with the stump," he says. "I walked fantastically well for an amputation above the knee." Feeling confident, the Cannizzaros returned to the West Coast. But, as Cannizzaro quickly learned, expenses, including medical costs, were much higher in California.

So, with an income below the poverty level, Steve reluctantly went back to the VA.

"In April," he recalls, "I thought, well, I'll go out to the veterans' hospital and see if I could get on their program for diabetics. I went out there and waited three to four hours. I finally saw the doctor and told him due to my very low income I would like to be able to get my insulin, my needles from the VA. I was told immediately that they would give it to me one time and that was it. They wasn't gonna give me any more."

For eight months, Cannizzaro carefully kept himself alive with the minimal supplies he had wrested from the VA. In December, his needles and medication gone, he was forced to go back to the hospital. He found the situation unchanged.

"At the time, I was drinking gallons of water. I thought, uh-oh, my sugar's really out of control. I just couldn't afford a private doctor. So instead of using the needle once, I'd clean it off and use it twice because it was very expensive. Living on that income, you have to be careful. And I'm still careful. Just because you get something for nothing, that doesn't mean you waste it."

Unable to obtain the needed supplies, and dejected and fearful for his health, Cannizzaro reluctantly reentered the VA system. After waiting four hours for a blood test, he was sent home. "I was very high-strung that day and breaking down and crying, due to the fact that my sugar level was so high."

By late afternoon, with no word from the VA and no longer able to contain his fears, Cannizzaro went to the VFW for help. "By that time, I was really broken up." Armed with a VFW representative, Cannizzaro was taken to the hospital admissions office, where the official on duty—first questioning Cannizzaro's reported difficulty in getting to see a doctor—admitted him for treatment. "Thank God I found somebody that really was interested in the patient," Cannizzaro says. "He suggested to the doctors to take my sugar count. It was very high, and they put me in the hospital. If it was left to the doctors, they woulda sent me home again."

Cannizzaro leans back in his seat for a moment and takes a deep breath. He is a gentle man with thick bushy eyebrows and gray hair with enough black still in it to make guessing his age difficult. He is wearing green checked pants and a yellow short-sleeve shirt that fits his stocky frame. On one foot is a white loafer. The other pants leg, empty, lies flat against the chair he is sitting in. He is surrounded by boxes in his apartment three blocks from the beach. He and Ruby are preparing to move back to Indiana again, and the green and yellow rugs are covered with string and wrapping paper.

Cannizzaro explains that while he was being treated in the hospital for diabetes, the doctors suggested that, even though it wasn't bothering him, it might be a good idea to have his stump revised—open it up, make sure all was well and refit the artificial leg.

"They told me it would be no problem and, anyway, when I was first operated on in 1969, the doctors said it wouldn't be a bad idea five, six years down the road to get it revised. Also, the doctor taking care of me for the diabetes was just great. So when she suggested the revision, I said okay. They did the revision. It was a success. Just beautiful. I was so happy with the whole thing."

And then the problems began.

"After I got out of the hospital, I started getting groin pains. I was coming back to prosthetics and they were cutting the socket down. They thought the difficulty was in the socket."

Examination confirmed the presence of a hernia. Readmitted to the hospital, he was assured that the problem was slight, requiring only an overnight stay for the simple operation. Three days later, Cannizzaro was finally wheeled into the operating room. "I was the last one scheduled," he says. "The doctor did six or seven that day and I was last because the problem was so slight, so minor. She said all I'd need was local anesthesia, that's all."

In the operating room, the doctor told her patient that he would be back in his room on the ward in twenty minutes. Cannizzaro told his wife he would call her then. "Dr. Y. said I'd feel the first cut. Just a little bit. You know how they talk to ya. So I felt the first cut, like she said. Then, after five or six minutes—I don't know, time goes fast like that—I heard her say, 'You're gonna have to put him all the way out.' So I went out."

Several hours later, not twenty minutes, Cannizzaro shook off the lingering effects of the general anesthetic. By then, his wife, waiting at home for the promised call, was frantic. She finally found her husband at midnight, some nine hours after he was rolled into the operating room—and after she threatened to call the police.

"They told her I was in the recovery room. But I was in the surgical intensive care unit," says Cannizzaro, an eighteen-hour-a-week volunteer at the hospital. "That was a damn lie." At six the next morning, Dr. Y. told Cannizzaro he would be discharged in twenty-four hours. Cannizzaro objected. The head doctor, called in for consultation, agreed with the patient. It was a fortunate decision.

Three days later, the stump swelled up. It didn't go down for a month. Nor did the pain. Finally, at the urging of a VA doctor sympathetic to Cannizzaro's plight, Cannizzaro went to an outside specialist. "He knew immediately what it was. 'You have lymphedema. They must have done something wrong to you.' He said they cut too deep and they cut the lymphatic glands. 'I'm only going by what I see.' "

Apparently, what he saw was correct. Cannizzaro was put back in the hospital.

"They did absolutely nothing for two months," he says. "Not a thing. No therapy. Nothing." Told by a hospital friend to get all his records because they did a "bum operation," Cannizzaro made a formal statement outlining what had happened.

"In the meantime, they're making it very miserable for me."

Eventually, Cannizzaro was invited to see Dr. H., the hospital's chief of staff. " 'Steve, we made a mistake here,' [Dr. H.] says to me. 'And I'm gonna tell you what they did wrong. They cut too low, and when they went to sew you back up, they ran the needle through the main artery, and when they went down to get that out, they cut the lymph gland. But we feel we can do something for you.' "

Nothing was done for eight weeks.

Finally, Cannizzaro was offered the opportunity to take a venogram, a highly dangerous procedure that Cannizzaro got them to admit would not help him in any way. It was strictly for the VA's benefit. Cannizzaro angrily went back to Dr. H. and demanded, "Fix me or pay me."

So far, they've done neither. Not only that, the VA has threatened to take away the compensation it agreed to award Cannizzaro because he left the hospital in worse shape than when he went in. So, from month to month, he and his wife were not sure how many groceries to buy, or whether they would be getting enough money to cover their outstanding checks. In addition, the letters Cannizzaro had friends and business associates send to the VA to prove that he was able to ambulate prior to the operation —somehow, he says, the letters have disappeared from his file.

Even the statement of the assistant chief, Rehabilitation Medicine, in Cannizzaro's hospital summary of November 8, 1977, is ignored.

The statement concludes, ". . . it is felt that there is probably a direct relationship between the surgical procedure and the development of the swelling in the stump. . . . The patient's disability has become chronic and his ability to ambulate with prosthesis has been markedly impaired. Absolute proof that the surgical procedure produced this result has not been established, but from a circumstantial standpoint there appears to be a direct causal relationship."

And Cannizzaro must also contend with the VA's publicly stated outrage that he complains too much to his congressional representatives!

None of which, of course, will ever get Cannizzaro out of the wheelchair he is now confined to and back walking again. "It's been agony," he says. "It's been upsetting to the wife to the point to where sometimes our life was very miserable together because of the strain that we had. We'd argue because of the pressure that was put on me to quit, just to give up, and get out of there. I was in the hospital more than two years total.

"They've never written to me, they've never said, 'We're sorry, Steve, that this has happened to you.' Instead, I get letters telling me that my money might be cut, taken away from me. And the doctor that operated on me? That disgusts me, too. I think the doctor should be reprimanded. Now, the doctor herself did not do it. It was a student doctor."

Because the Long Beach VA is affiliated with the nearby medical school at the University of California at Irvine, many "student doctors" get part of their education at the hospital. Medical students, residents, and interns, still in training and nominally under the supervision of a licensed and certified physician, all rotate through the largest general medical and surgical facility in the VA system. And it is no coincidence that Cannizzaro's operation, presented as safe and surefire, was proposed while he was hospitalized for something else. And it is no accident that the operation apparently wasn't even close to being necessary. Cannizzaro was, basically, sweet-talked into allowing it.

"They certainly were real nice to me before they operated. The way it turned out, I've wondered about that," Cannizzaro says.

At a teaching hospital, material for the students must constantly be provided. For the year ending in September 1978, for example, a total of 4,672 operations of all kinds were performed at Long Beach. An incredible 96 percent (4,476) were done by residents. Staff accounted for a mere 196 operations during that period.

The overwhelming number of operations (2,056) were of a general surgery nature, of the type Cannizzaro was subjected to. One thousand nine hundred eighty-three (96 percent) had a resident's signature on them. The percentages are similar nationwide.

The Long Beach–Irvine relationship is regarded as a "very important resource to our educational program," Dr. Stanley Vandenoort, dean, UC-Irvine Medical School, candidly testified in 1974 before Senator Alan Cranston's Subcommittee on Health and Hospitals of the Committee on Veterans' Affairs. "It is pretty obvious with four hundred medical students and six hundred twenty projected residents, and with a faculty of several hundred, that [the medical school's own] two-hundred-bed hospital isn't going to fulfill very much of our educational program."

Most postgraduate and "hands-on" medical training in this country is done at those nonprivate facilities where patients are generally poor or otherwise unable to afford private care, a characteristic of the large majority of VA patients who are then lumped into the "welfare" category—and treated accordingly.

Because these patients have nowhere else to go, they are less likely to object to not-completely-trained physicians administering medical care to them. Frequently, as is true of the VA, they are not even told the training status of those operating on them. Private hospitals are much more circumspect and restrictive in their policies. Their patients can demand the real, completely educated thing—and they can afford, with insurance or cash, to take their business elsewhere.

As Terry G. Holder, a paralyzed marine and an active former official in the California Paralyzed Veterans Association, told the Subcommittee on Health and Hospitals in 1974,

Because of medical school affiliation with the VA, patients are receiving unnecessary operations (or, at least, are being pressured into agreeing to such operations) so that interns and residents, from medical schools, can get experience—at the patient's expense—in certain medical areas where they actually have live "guinea pigs" to work on. (I was told by one doctor that I would need a "TUR"—transurethral resection—to "help the bladder.")

Good heavens! My bladder is working very well for a paraplegic and, even though [Dr. E., a urologist] also tried to talk me into letting the resident doctor operate, I refused.

Dr. Y., who told Cannizzaro his "simple" hernia operation was nothing to worry about, was a resident in surgery when the events leading to the malpractice suit took place.

"She's a very good doctor," says Dr. H., the chief of staff who admitted to Cannizzaro that a "mistake" had occurred. "She was one of our best. The fact that a suit may be won does not mean that a physician is guilty.

"First of all, there's no proof, in any scientific sense, that Steve's outcome had been the result of some malfeasance on the part of the physician. A supposition is about as far as it would go. On the other hand, at the same time there is no way of proving that what was done didn't have an influence on the outcome. So it's a matter of giving the patient the benefit of the doubt.

"It doesn't necessarily mean that the surgeon did anything wrong. But in the course of surgery any number of things can happen, and the outcome can be adverse even if nobody's at fault. In many, many surgical situations that's true."

But, Dr. H. maintains, "there's no question" that the medical school affiliation "has brought about an improvement in patient care."

All Steve Cannizzaro knows is that when he entered that VA hospital he could walk. And that when he left, he was in a wheelchair.

"When I was first amputated, the [non-VA] doctor guaranteed me that I would be wearing an artificial limb," Cannizzaro says, his usually quiet voice rising perceptibly at the injustice. "So I did have a future a little bit, of being able to walk, of being a man again. Now, they took that privilege away from me, which I'll never get back again.

"Actually, I'm in worse condition now than I was when they

amputated the first time. Hard as it is to believe, they amputated another leg."

Cannizzaro takes a deep breath. "They actually amputated an artificial limb," he says. "Can you beat that?"

It is four-thirty on a dreary and humid Friday afternoon, and federal employees, heading in a well-worn frenzy for the rush-hour subways and buses, are leaving the building in animated clots of fagged humanity.

Downstairs in the lobby of the Veterans Administration's New York Regional Office, a decrepit hulk of a structure symbolic of the system it fitfully represents, two dirt-filmed social realism wall murals funnel the hundreds of workers from the busy bank of operator-run elevators toward the street and the weekend.

One of the paintings, both of which tower some thirty feet over the homeward-bound commuters, is a frieze-dried rendering of a white-coated figure supporting a man in civilian clothes who has his left pants leg rolled up to reveal an artificial limb. The appendage is being sympathetically fitted by another figure in white bending down to help.

Behind all three is a kneeling soldier, his expression fixed with a serious, faraway look. He is holding a machine gun cradled in his right arm, barbed wire encircling the ground around him. On the other side of the monumental canvas, behind the three figures, is a green army van with a bold red cross on its side. The vehicle is parked in front of several buildings, including factory smokestacks symbolic of a vital industry and economy. A crutch lies discarded behind the crouching white-garbed figures.

On the opposite wall, in the foreground, a well-groomed civilian with crisp white shirt, rolled-up sleeves, and a tie—all protected by a white apron—is sitting at a small lathe. His right arm, working on the machine, is fitted with a hook.

Standing unobtrusively behind his left shoulder and guiding his (good) left arm as it works the apparatus, is a woman in white with an Occupational Therapy patch on her left sleeve. Behind her, in the dim light, a determined GI scans the skies through an antiaircraft battery, a ship sails in the near grayness. In back of the lathe operator's left shoulder a new car, 1940s vintage, sits. It has whitewall tires. In the distance are bold, sturdy, aggressive industrial structures.

Both paintings, executed by David Lax in 1952, are overwhelmed with dark blue brooding skies.

Farther along the walls are official printed signs: "All persons must sign the register" and "All packages and/or brief cases subject to inspection."

Like the murals, the signs are ignored.

On the seventh floor, where health care is offered to eligible veterans, paint is peeling from the sides of the patient waiting area. Tom Sherwood's office suite down the hall has nicely maintained rust-colored wall-to-wall carpeting, wood veneer wall panels, and new-looking furniture.

The area is separated from the medical and surgical outpatient reception section by two heavy tan and black doors with shatter-resistant chicken-wire glass. Sherwood, a slightly balding black man with a goatee, sits behind his desk in an inner room. He is eager to talk, and when he does, the words glide out with feeling.

"Unfortunately for some people, I am one of those who is very much into patient care," Sherwood says. "Patient care is basic to me."

Sherwood, an executive-level employee, looks around the office, and tells a story.

"I was on the ward floor and I saw a senior resident with his flock of PG-Ones [first-year residents] around him, doing his head trip. You could see it was a head trip. I've worked with doctors twenty-two years, I know what I'm talking about. Okay, he's teaching and I arrived to watch him confront a patient in a wheelchair.

"And the patient was begging, begging in his chair, begging this doctor not to take any more blood from him. " 'You've stuck me, doctor, for eight days in a row, except Sunday. Eight days in a row, and I think you're doing the same thing now, and you won't tell me why you're taking this blood and you're taking it out of the same arm. I'm bleeding from these punctures.'

"The doctor looked at his students and they were terrified by that because they knew it was wrong.

" 'I'm the doctor,' he says to the man in the wheelchair, 'and I know what you need. I know what's good for you. Now, if you don't like that, then you can get out, and I'll discharge you tomorrow if you don't let me take this blood.'

"I wept. I mean, I was shocked. Here I was, a registered nurse who had worked in intensive care units and had seen all kinds of stuff. And this was beyond me. I said to myself, be cool, be cool. Don't get into this righteous bag, just be very levelheaded about this. And I said, on the other hand, I'm on the staff and I have a responsibility to say something.

"I asked the doctor, very nicely, 'Doctor, could I see you on one side just for a few minutes?'

" 'Oh! Can't you see I'm busy? You see my students. I'm teaching. Who are you? Who are you?'

"I said, 'I'm on the director's staff.'

" 'Well, I have no time for you. I've got no time for you.' And he just took off with his embarrassed flock.

"All right? I said to myself if this is an example of what happens in this fucking hospital . . . I got downstairs to the director, my immediate superior, and the chief of staff, and I explained this incident, and I wrote it all up for them.

"I got a negative attitude, like I was wrong for saying that this hospital belongs to this patient.

"The chief of staff asked me for my report. I found out later from an administrator that he tore it up as soon as I left his office. He tore it up and then said, 'This guy's a troublemaker.' "

Tom Sherwood, forty-four, perhaps a "troublemaker," is no ordinary critic of the VA. He can't be dismissed as some disgruntled vet whom a quick Thorazine fix will straighten out. He's not some punk newspaper reporter with an ax to grind and a news hole to fill. Nor is he an addled politician hoping to make it through one more election on the stooped backs of an alcoholic veteran or two.

Tom Sherwood, articulate, candid, is special assistant to the director in charge of the out-patient clinic at the Manhattan VA Medical Center, one of the largest facilities in the agency, with a budget of $72 million. He is also head of the Prosthetics–Sensory Aid Services, the third largest service of its type, with a $700,000 budget. Sherwood is, in short, one of the top four people at the center.

He is also one of the few in the system who, given the opportunity, have the ability and foresight to save it and reenergize it as a vital, vibrant health-care provider. One chief of service calls him the conscience of the hospital.

The Manhattan VA hospital itself is a mammoth multistory skyscraper about a twenty-minute walk across town from Sherwood and the regional office. The lobby there, where the end-of-the-day rush has already abated, is mostly empty. There are no overbearing murals to greet visitors, only a warning: "Please have your ID ready to be checked by hospital police."

Right next to that is a large plaque: "Veterans Administration Hospital—Erected 1950."

Sitting in the waiting area on the street level, one gets a feel for the flow of activity. Several seats are occupied by people gazing absently out toward the traffic creeping home up First Avenue. At the center, a half-dozing black man who looks to be in his mid-forties is approached by a woman in white.

She is obviously going off her tour of duty for the day. She apparently remembers the man as a patient and asks what is wrong. At first, there is no response. Then, slowly awakening and clearly in pain, he moans softly in response to her attentions.

"Didn't they take care of you?" she asks.

The man moans.

"Did they discharge you? Do you have any place to go?"

He moans again, tears welling up in his eyes.

The woman, concerned, rises and tells the man to stay where he is. She rushes off in the direction of the elevators. Five minutes later, she returns with a physician.

Tall and dressed in surgical greens with a matching hair net, he firmly and comfortingly takes the man's unsteady arm and guides him back to the elevators and, presumably, the treatment wards, which perhaps he should not have been allowed to leave to begin with.

The lady in white exits through the glass doors and heads home.

VA officials will, when pressed, acknowledge lapses in medical care and innocently blame them on the unavoidable pitfalls of a very large system, the same one whose size, they say, allows for the economies of scale that bring quality care in the first place. "Complaints are bound to happen in an organization that big," says California Senator Alan Cranston, who insists that the VA is "much better" than it was ten years ago.

"It happens everywhere. Some personnel are careless, some don't care," adds the former chairman of the Senate Veterans' Affairs Committee. "Or an administrator may not be doing well. It's unavoidable. They're human beings and human beings aren't perfect. One of the problems is the VA's vastness and difficulty in implanting a substantial feeling of concern and sensitivity. It's hard to ensure that you will get people to act with sympathy and concern. That's something that pervades and hurts. It's an ever-lasting problem."

"I'm sure some of these [negative] reports are valid," echoes A. M. Willis, Jr., for the last six years staff director of the House Veterans' Affairs Committee, "but there are two sides."

Like the current chairman of the committee, Ray Roberts, and another one before him, Olin "Tiger" Teague, Willis is from Texas, a self-professed "LBJ man." Outspoken and, like his hero from the Pedernales, just this side of fully civilized, Willis punctuates his opinions with down-home, country-boy clearings of his gastrointestinal tract.

"Veterans are human beings [just as, presumably Cranston's VA employees are] and human beings have a tendency to see (phsst) things their own way sometimes. But I wouldn't go so far as to say someone is lying when I don't know he's lying. Maybe some of them had a hard time (pooot) with his life in the service.

"He starts rehashing it. Convinced he's been mistreated. I don't know. But I can tell you we pay a lot of claims we don't owe (phoo-zzst)."

Still, complaints should be followed up, says lawyer Dean Phillips, a special assistant to Max Cleland and a Silver Star Vietnam paratrooper. "You can't just wave your hand and say, oh, c'mon, now, the VA is responsive to every veteran who ever files a claim. You have an agency with a twenty-one-billion-dol-lar-a-year annual budget, fifty-seven regional offices, a hundred and seventy-two medical centers, ten million claims for benefits a year.

"Say the VA did an excellent job in ninety-nine percent of those contacts with those ten million claims for benefits. Excellent job in ninety-nine percent. That means a hundred thousand fuck-ups. Right? So I think you gotta check it out. Find out if it's an incident misconstrued by the veteran or the individual person at the VA.

"Or find out if there's a pattern, if there's consistent complaints about the same facility, particularly if they're verifiable ones. Then you start looking at making some changes. It just depends. Each thing's gotta be looked at individually on its merits."

Cleland himself admits to "isolated incidents. Occasionally we make mistakes."

For some, however, that's not good enough.

On October 25, 1979, Veterans of Foreign Wars National Commander Howard Vander Clute, Jr., told a joint House-Senate Veterans' Affairs Committee hearing on the VA that "we of the VFW believe that even if one veteran who served our great nation on active duty in the armed forces is denied needed medical care or hospitalization by the Veterans Administration, then that agency is remiss in its duty to our veterans, if not derelict in its duty."

Sometimes the dereliction is more insidious.

Far removed from the brooding murals and ignored patients of a busy city, Durham, North Carolina, smells tobacco-sweet in the glittering early morning sunshine. Soon, it will heat up to the day's rhythms of a progressive southern community, where a smile and a handshake are valued among equals.

This community's VA Medical Center sits in comfortable proximity to Duke University's prestigious private medical school.

The early sunlight shows off the well-kept waiting areas whose seats, covered with stylish fabric, are actually soft and restful. A seashell collection is on display in a nearby glass case. A visitor has the impression that the facility, a five-story red-brick building, is much newer than its announced thirty years. Its physical appearance is reflected in the upbeat, caring attitudes obvious in staff, administration, and patients.

It's an agreeable place.

But there are problems.

Dr. Paul Schafer, chief of Thoracic Surgery at the Washington, D.C., VA Medical Center and a researcher in cell biology, is president of the National Association of VA Physicians (NAVAP), a five-year-old group that represents more than 6,000 full-time physicians out of the approximately 18,000 (including residents) currently employed by the VA. He believes the VA health-care delivery system is in a state of crisis, and he lays the blame, at least in part, on the nation's medical schools affiliated with VA hospitals throughout the country.

The vehicle for the affiliation, and the subsequent consternation, is something called the Deans' Committee, a creation in 1946 of Drs. Paul Hawley and Paul Magnuson during the halcyon days of General Bradley. The committee, composed of faculty members of the affiliated school, recommends to the VA the medical staff to be hired. Though progressive and farsighted in concept, the process quickly became abused in execution, and all sorts of animosities and suspicions have arisen through the years.

A major complaint is that the committee, which usually consists of powerful, aggressive doctors, tends to dominate the relationship, to the detriment of the VA and the veteran.

"In some instances, the medical school has been running the VA hospital," acknowledges Rep. Ray Roberts, chairperson of the House Veterans' Affairs Committee. "But we can't operate properly without the affiliation."

In 1976, NAVAP's Schafer, a VA physician for sixteen years, made a weeklong site visit to the Durham VA. As part of the VA's Systematic External Review Program (SERP), the regularly scheduled inspection, conducted by a team of career VA professionals, is intended to augment the biannual quality surveys done by the Joint Commission on the Accreditation of Hospitals.

The visit, described in locked VA central office files, still visibly upsets Schafer, who personally refused to identify the facility.

"The absolute nadir was reached when I sat down privately

with one of the chief surgery residents," he says with a great deal of agitation. "This is a guy who had been there seven years. He was just finishing his training. And we go over all the nice things. He's very polite to me. He's seen me several times. He knows my background.

"He's obviously been briefed on things we've been saying and he said, 'Dr. Schafer, you know, we're not a big city like yours. We don't have any D.C. General Hospital. We don't have anything like Chicago's Cook County Hospital.' And he went on through Bellevue, and he reeled off a whole bunch of them. Then he said— Schafer's voice rises here—"he said, 'This is our charity hospital. And, by God, these veterans are just awful lucky to be getting such good free care.'

"Well, I looked at this guy and I said, 'Young man, after seven years, how can you possibly say that to me? I know, charitably, you're reflecting only what your supervisors, through these seven years, have projected to you, because that must be their view, too.'

"He said, 'Sure, we all feel that way.' I said, 'Well, I'm going to tell you something that I want you to remember till your dying day. Every one of these patients in this hospital has already prepaid it in coin like you never will get from your most affluent practice independently. And you should be goddamned ashamed of yourself for having such an attitude.' "

Schafer points out that he reported that conversation "almost verbatim" in the exit conference, the meeting the inspection team holds with the top officials of the facility once the visit is completed.

"You meet with the hospital administrator, the chief of staff, the chiefs of service around a nice big conference table in a plush, paneled room. I told them exactly what I had experienced. They weren't too surprised. They knew it existed. But they also knew that the Deans' Committee in that relationship was so powerful they couldn't do a goddamn thing about it."

Later, Schafer reports, the SERP team sat in on a Deans' Committee meeting. "It was a charade," says Schafer, whose wavy, graying hair reaches almost to the collar of his long white lab coat. "Hell, the VA types might as well have been puppets."

According to some Durham VA people, the string-pulling is mutual and evenly distributed.

"The relationship here is excellent. The [physical] closeness is what makes this thing work," insists Burley McGraw, the twenty-eight-year VA employee who is the administrative assistant to the associate chief of staff. "There's not a sense of malicious rivalry. In fact, it's just the opposite," he says, then adds, "Of course, you don't hire a Ph.D. if Duke doesn't want him. You just don't do that."

B. Fred Brown is the hospital's amiable, open director. He, too, appears content with his role vis-à-vis Duke.

"State universities have a different personality than private medical schools," he explains. "Duke is aggressive, high quality, on the cutting edge of the field of medicine. It's got the resources and it's pushing hard. Some people interpret that to be dominant. My own feeling is that our VA patients would not be getting quality health care if Duke wasn't pushing to bring it on the line. I think we're very fortunate.

"You give up a little autonomy," Brown, twenty-one years with the VA and head of Durham since January 1979, continues. "I do not consider that to be dominant. If as director you want to sit back and give it to them, you can do that and the school will fill the vacuum. But there's no way we would be doing open-heart surgery, kidney dialysis, neurosurgery if we weren't affiliated with the medical school. We just wouldn't have them."

Both the Manhattan VA and the Durham VA are affiliated with a medical school—large, powerful medical-education juggernauts—New York University and Duke University, respectively.

All told, in 1979, 136 of the system's 172 hospitals and thirty-eight out-patient clinic facilities were formally affiliated with 104 medical schools. Fifty-eight dental schools were affiliated with ninety hospitals. During 1978, a total of 97,272 trainees, up more than 1,500 from 1977, went through the system. The numbers included 22,561 medical residents in 1,432 specialty resident programs, 19,550 medical students, 29,540 nursing students, and 1,031 dental students.

The medical schools receive millions of dollars each year

through this arrangement, some $2.5 billion in the past two decades.

In fact, however, the entire affiliation arrangement, which basically allows the VA to bring medical trainees into a government facility for educational purposes, is legally and professionally questionable. But with billions of dollars and cheap medical care at stake (doctors in training receive far less salary than do full-time trained physicians), not too many people care to rock the gold-laden boat.

In 1946, during the glory days of General Bradley and amid the prevailing optimism that, finally, a health-care system second to none would indeed blossom for America's veterans, the VA, anxious to lure the prestigious medical schools at almost any cost, issued what many believe is its single most important document. Coauthored by the number one and number two men in the newly minted Department of Medicine and Surgery (DM&S), Drs. Hawley and Magnuson, the document was preceded by a letter sent to the deans of the nation's medical schools. The letter asked for their "consent to willingness to cooperate" in an arrangement whereby the schools and selected VA hospitals would share facilities and staff for the purpose of training medical personnel. The letter was followed up with an official agency statement, Policy Memorandum No. 2, "Policy in Association of Veterans Hospitals with Medical Schools."

The document is unique, both for the circumstances of its issuance as well as its contents. Contrary to federal regulations, the plan was never printed in the VA's formally published bulletins, a mandated practice that allows public input prior to the implementation of proposed interpretations of existing law. No written contract, legal wording, or mutual signatories accompanied the execution of the arrangement, unheard of in the bureaucratic world of government business.

Additionally, Policy Memorandum No. 2, which, because of its informality came to be known as the "Gentleman's Agreement," was a unilateral statement proffered by the VA without the knowledge or consent of Congress. Benjamin Lewis, in his exhaustive but not overly critical examination of the VA's affiliation history, calls the plan "atypical for government" and politely excuses the casualness about legal amenities. It was a strange departure for that bastion of bureaucracy and a mother lode for the medical school community, though the deans and other medical administrators were slow at first to realize its potential. Its full significance, and the impact of what amounted to untapped wealth, came into even sharper focus as the medical institutions hit the fiscal skids. Never before had a government agency so willingly given up to a private entity the power to determine its internal employment policies and overall hiring circumstances. It is the only example in the federal government in which private individuals are allowed, indeed encouraged, to assert de facto control over the staffing priorities, job status, and qualifications of ostensibly public employees.

By law, the Deans' Committees, forbidden from having VA employees as voting members, make "nominations" to the VA for approval. It is the contention of many in the VA, as well as of veterans and some medical school personnel, that the schools have actually been given a blank check to run the affiliated VA hospitals. And, they add, the blank check is not legally redeemable.

The role of the hospital director, the federal employee responsible for the running of a publicly financed facility, was reduced to that of a domesticated houseboy taking orders from the private sector's master by virtue of the provision that he, or she, "will cooperate with the Deans' Committee, bringing to its attention any dereliction of duty on the part of its nominees." The director can't even fire, much less refuse to hire, some of the people who work under him!

Even the overall mission of the VA hospital system is changed when a school agrees to affiliate. No longer is health care of the veteran the overriding concern and priority. According to the VA's own interpretation of its responsibilities, and stated nowhere in Policy Memorandum No. 2 or elsewhere, DM&S will "complement the programs of affiliated medical and dental schools and *adjust its activities to insure completion of its curricular* responsibilities within the affiliation." (Italics added.)

All this authority is derived, the VA claims, from P.L.293, which established the Department of Medicine and Surgery and permitted the VA to affiliate with medical schools. The Deans' Committee, however, was solely a creature of Policy Memorandum No. 2. In the end, critics insist, the memorandum, meant to enhance the quality of veterans' health care and provide for the training of medical specialists in an atmosphere of mutual sharing and trust, became a tool for the aggrandizement of the medical school establishment at the expense of the veteran patient.

"I think," says Dr. Schafer, "if any public-interest groups want to hire counsel and go into court, this [arrangement] would be found to be illegal. There is no way any court of law in this country would countenance it, but we accept it in everyday practice. In effect, the Deans' Committee is determining the professional staffing in federal institutions, which means the way public tax monies are being spent. And that is just a basic violation of everything we know about proprieties between public and private sectors."

"VA medicine has a fuzzy legal basis," agrees Oliver Meadows, the former congressional staff director who "produced" all those media horror stories in 1970. "It [affiliation] is a relationship we backed into. It certainly wasn't legally sanctioned. Of course, it was generally accepted and recognized by everyone, and the VA couldn't get along without it. But it wasn't legal."

The Veterans Administration's general counsel, Guy McMichael III, insists there is no question about the legality or propriety of the VA–medical school relationship. The Deans' Committees "do not appoint VA physicians," he notes, "nor do they have 'veto' power over VA appointments of its physicians." He says the committees' role is "expressly limited." Aside from the fact that nowhere does this language appear in Title 38 of the U.S. Code, the legislative backbone of VA authority, the *reality* of it is also questioned by McMichael's own boss—Max Cleland.

"The affiliation is a unique mixture," Cleland asserts, "but where we get hurt is if that hospital director and that chief of staff don't stand up for us. We have to watch our leadership in the field because they can easily be blown out, in some stations; easily blown out by a medical school. But we try not to cave in to that type of thing, blackmail on the part of the medical school."

Sometimes, says Cleland, keeping the VA from being overrun and dominated by the schools "can be very difficult. It depends on the leadership of DM&S from top to bottom."

Thus, while Title 38 does give legal authority to the Deans' Committee, as pointed out by McMichael, it does not explicitly define the committee's mandate. In addition, and important to the understanding of the VA's historically haphazard relationship to the schools, even the cover of law was not bestowed upon the Deans' Committee by Congress until 1965—a full twenty years after it had become established VA procedure!

"It is unfortunate that something that has been so good is now beginning to be abused," Schafer says. "It's part of the economy of our times. The medical schools and universities are feeling a horrible money pinch. That means now they are leaner, more aggressive, more avaricious. The pendulum is now swinging to the point where they are using the system. To the extent they do use it, then all those good things that they did bring to the relationship will begin to depreciate. The Hawley-Magnuson plan signaled a promising future."

The future has arrived, all right, but somewhere along the way the signals have turned from promising to sour. The extremes to which the medical schools have taken the lucrative affiliation route are nowhere more transparent than at the Philadelphia VA. There, two powerful medical institutions, the Medical College of Pennsylvania and the University of Pennsylvania School of Medicine, vie for Uncle Sam's dollars. The schools are so desperate for the largesse that they have worked out a unique arrangement. Incredible as it might seem to the average Joe on the wards, each school has its own service, so that at the Philadelphia VA there are *two* medical services, *two* surgery services, *two* psychiatry services, and so on.

Instead of the quality of care being twice as effective, as one might hope, if not expect, there have been significant problems.

Outlining deteriorating patient services at the facility, including abusive doctors and students, long waiting lines, and below-standard care, Robert Vogel, an official of the Pennsylvania American Legion, told a congressional committee in 1977, ". . . we have concern about two medical schools in one Veterans Administration hospital, each maintaining separate services with separate chiefs. Our concerns center around added building space, and competition between the two schools, causing jealousy and greed which in turn could downgrade the quality of medical care to the veteran."

Other testimony at the hearings concludes, "It appears that many feel that the hospital would run smoother if it were affiliated with only one school."

In Philadelphia, medical schools know a good thing when they see it. Sometimes, they know it even when they don't see it.

In the early 1960s, the College of Medicine at Ohio State University declared publicly that it was affiliated, through its Deans' Committee, with the Chillicothe VA hospital. Unfortunately, the hospital itself was at the same time telling Congress that it was not affiliated with any medical school. Because no formal contractual arrangements were ever made—entirely typical of VA affiliation policy until recently—the medical school was able to trade on the name of the VA by falsely extending its list of training sites to entice prospective postgraduate students to its program. In addition, the VA seemed reluctant to offend the educational institution by suggesting that, since the affiliation had been inactive for a number of years, perhaps an officially sanctioned severance should take place.

Medical school officials are quick to extol the virtues of affiliations, nonetheless. Sometimes, they say, it is the VA that acts unilaterally.

"The [San Francisco] VA recently hired some staff without telling or consulting with the medical school. They just did it without us," bemusedly complains Dr. William Hamilton, chief of staff, chairman of the Department of Anesthesiology and a member of the Deans' Committee at the VA-affiliated University of California–San Francisco medical school.

It is generally regarded as perhaps the best affiliation agreement in the VA system.

"I've seen VAs with and without medical school affiliations," Hamilton says simply. "There is superior health care with an affiliation." One reason it is superior is the caliber of the staff, both the mature doctor as well as the younger residents and interns, according to Hamilton.

"We work very closely with the VA," says Dr. Lloyd Smith, chairman of the UCSF Department of Medicine, a member of the Deans' Committee and a veteran of the Korean War. He suggests that UCSF is in an excellent position to attract the best new physicians in the United States. With tight supervision, the patient benefits in the process.

"Young, bright students bring up other views. They'll often turn up some interesting things that we'll overlook. If I were seriously ill, I wouldn't want to be anywhere where there were no interns and residents. They're very sharp in handling medical emergencies, and they tend to be more competent than older doctors. The young physician is up to date on all the latest ideas and technology."

"We're so closely affiliated with the medical school, it adds a lot of quality," concurs Dr. Sandy Kiser, a psychiatric consultant to the Dallas VA. "You can't get a quality person unless you get him a university affiliation. Otherwise, you'll get a typical VA doc who shuffles papers.

"The VA is so bulky, so unwieldy and inflexible," Kiser adds, "that getting care to the patient means getting around the rules. It's really a shame. But there's no question the quality of care rises when the VA is affiliated with medical schools. It's the maze of forced regulations that impedes the ability of the VA."

Kiser's boss at the University of Texas's Southwestern Medical School in Dallas agrees. "The VA grows with a lot of pitching of the ship," says Dr. Kenneth Altshuler, chairman of the Department of Psychiatry. "It's clear, though, that an affiliation alters the thing from a Civil Service post to something vital."

One thing that is not vital, everyone agrees, is the hospital with no medical school connection. "The non-affiliated VA hospital is usually not staffed to provide the most sophisticated techniques available," understates a 1974 University of California–San Francisco Health Policy Program report. "It cannot provide a comprehensive range of services to the patient."

The study, *The Role of the Veterans Administration Medical System in the American Health Care Enterprise,* was commissioned and paid for by the VA.

Citing an unnamed California VA chief of staff as its source, the 156-page document notes that "although not all VA hospitals are of equal quality, the veteran may not be aware of differences among them or the *risks associated* with such differences. . . . The isolated VA hospital may find itself in the position of placing the *unsuspecting patient in needless risk by performing a procedure of which it is only marginally capable.*" (Italics added.)

The specter of criminal negligence, not to mention moral and ethical bankruptcy, apparently caused few VA administrators any sleepless nights in their pursuit of health-care excellence. Nor did it seem to arouse congressional committees or veterans' service organizations to incensed action.

If some hospitals are placing patients—veterans—at risk, a reasonable assumption would be that those facilities be identified. To do otherwise is indecent and criminal. Not only didn't the VA name those hospitals, but the agency went blithely along its way crowing that, across the board, the nation's veterans were all getting care second to none!

One such hospital was identified, but its identity was buried on page 396 of a special report on the quality of VA patient care undertaken by the House Veterans' Affairs Committee and issued October 26, 1974, just three months after the Health Policy Program paper was released. The hospital was the Livermore VA, the very same facility constructed on the grounds whose price was so obligingly inflated by Colonel Forbes fifty years earlier.

The anger of the survey team comes through at the outset of its report. So does the outrage.

It is [our] general opinion that the level of the quality of care at VA Livermore is inadequate. There is also a consensus . . . that the professional competence of some of the physicians on the rolls of this hospital is lacking.

What has been done well in one area, the physical plant, is completely offset by the inadequacies of the professional staff. Except for the Chief of Medicine (who intends to leave, he says), the doctors tend to be aged and ailing, like their patients.

They have no leadership, there is no ongoing program of medical education, and they will escape rendering poor medical care only by assiduously avoiding the acceptance of cases beyond their capabilities to adequately diagnose and treat. . . . The Chief of Medicine cited several instances where members of the staff had not adequately met the needs of certain patients with bleeding conditions, pulmonary insufficiency, and gastrointestinal bleeding.

We can leave it to the imagination—and the conscience of the VA—to estimate how many American veterans, safely home from the battlefield, died or had their condition worsened after they went in, suffering, to seek help at Livermore and other, similar VA medical centers.

The VA, of course, made no effort to warn veterans away from these houses of, literally, ill repute. (Very much in character, however, it did gingerly let the public know that parts of the Livermore facility were not built to withstand earthquakes, and accordingly reduced the number of beds there.)

Nor did the VA have the ethical resources to make public the identities of those hospitals that were found lacking—as well as those found to be superior—in another agency-sponsored study, this one published in 1977. The National Academy of Sciences (NAS) survey, ordered by the ninety-third Congress in 1973 at the request of the VA, took three years to complete and cost taxpayers $6 million. Much of the data was gathered at about the same time the Health Policy Program and the Livermore materials were being put together.

The NAS work, severely criticized by the VA and its allies in Congress as "overgeneralizing," made thirty-seven recommendations. The VA disagreed completely with fourteen of them and in a limited way with another ten. Among its conclusions was the belief, backed by statistics, that patients in nonaffiliated hospitals tended to get poor or inadequate care. The same conclusion was drawn relative to psychiatric hospitals in the system.

In its final report, NAS discussed the quality of acute in-patient care in twenty-one randomly selected VA general hospitals. Identifying them only with a secret code number, NAS labeled five of them "Outstanding," thirteen "Adequate," and three "Inadequate." Hospitals rated inadequate had low medical staff-to-patient ratios, and no interns or residents. NAS also ranked the hospitals on five different measures of the process of care: completeness of the initial examination, follow-up on abnormalities detected, appropriateness of tests or treatments, patient education, and continuity of care after discharge.

Again, those facilities listed as inadequate fell at the low end of the ranking, as did some rated adequate.

In addition, the NAS team, which involved health-care professionals from all over the country, evaluated the medical services of six psychiatric hospitals. It found three to be inadequate in the overall quality of in-patient care delivered. Two others were rated adequate as chronic-care facilities, but with "management of acute medical problems considered beyond the clinical capabilities of the current medical staffs." Further, "Higher mortality rates and very low volumes of surgery were observed in psychiatric hospitals."

In total, five of the six psychiatric facilities evaluated had inadequate ability to take care of serious medical problems.

While the VA has made some changes recommended in the report—surgery, for example, has virtually disappeared from nonaffiliated psychiatric hospitals—it has never made public the names of the hospitals and their rankings. Thus, veterans and their families, some of whom, presumably, have already suffered medical abuse in poorly rated hospitals, will have to continue taking the risk that the facility in which hospitalization occurs is capable of caring for its patients. Conversely, veterans are prevented from making an informed choice about high-quality care for the same reasons. They have not been given the basic information that would allow them to decide for themselves where to go for help.

Although the VA (and, for that matter, NAS) still refuses to release the names of the hospitals in the report, it is possible to determine which ones they are.

The following, from congressional and VA sources, is the first general public listing of the twenty-seven facilities, along with the affiliated (A) or nonaffiliated (NA) status of each one.

Twenty-one general hospitals:

Bay Pines, Florida (NA); Durham, North Carolina (A); Fort Wayne, Indiana (NA); Iron Mountain, Michigan (NA); Leavenworth, Kansas (A); Long Beach, California (A); Madison, Wisconsin (A); Marlin, Texas (A); Memphis, Tennessee (A); Minneapolis, Minnesota (A); New Orleans, Louisiana (A); New York, New York (A); Philadelphia, Pennsylvania (A); Phoenix, Arizona (NA); Portland, Oregon (A); Salem, Virginia (A); Sepulveda, California (A); Shreveport, Louisiana (A); Sioux Falls, South Dakota (A); Tampa, Florida (A); West Roxbury, Massachusetts (A).

The six psychiatric hospitals:

Brentwood, Los Angeles, California (A); Chillicothe, Ohio (NA); Downey, Chicago, Illinois (A—now a general hospital); Murfreesboro, Tennessee (A); Northampton, Massachusetts (A); Waco, Texas (A—was not affiliated when study was done).

But an affiliation, despite all the ballyhoo, tub-thumping, and occasional statistics, is by no means an ironclad guarantee of decent health care. Sometimes, in fact, it is a red flag of warning.

At Durham, for example, medical residents on the wards determine who will be admitted based on the residents' own personal medical-training interests rather than the needs of the patient, according to testimony presented by a VFW official at a July 25, 1977, hearing before the Subcommittee on Medical Facilities and Benefits of the House Committee on Veterans' Affairs. It is a charge heard frequently and, in this instance, one not directly denied by the then-director of VA Durham.

"The schools are always looking for 'good' teaching cases," says Jeffrey Prottas, a Harvard professor who studied the VA.

Elsewhere in North Carolina, patient benefits accruing to the veteran are equally questionable.

Berimer Nelson, wounded in combat and recently retired from a career in the marines, tried to get help at the Fayetteville VA. He doesn't go there anymore, and it's not only because on several occasions he's waited eight hours only to be told by the pharmacist that they didn't have the medication his VA physician had prescribed for him.

"It just appears to me that they bounce you around from doctor to doctor. No one tells you anything and it's very frustrating. It appears that they're trying to give the interns practice. And after the end of the day, they tell you to go home. Nothing."

Ironically, the director of the Fayetteville VA, B. E. Phillips, in his statement to the subcommittee, inadvertently lent support to the accusations.

"As valuable as it is to us, our affiliation [with the University of North Carolina] does create a whole new set of demands which are taxing our existing resources to the maximum. I am certain that as the affiliation continues to emerge, we will not be able to satisfy the obligations of the hospital to the university and to our patients without additional monetary support for staff, educational space, and learning resources."

More to the point, however, it might serve health-care delivery better if educational arrangements were reduced or, at the very least, residents and interns were screened and supervised more scrupulously.

"When I worked at the Bronx VA as a lab technician, I used to go in and watch the autopsies that were being done in the autopsy room next door," remembers Dr. Howard Berliner, now an assistant professor of health policy at the NYU Graduate School of Public Administration. "The surgical residents were rotated through the autopsy room as part of their pathology training. They didn't want to do that. That to them was not real medicine. They weren't keeping someone alive. They were just cutting up someone dead.

"A lot of them used to get stoned and then go in and, you know, really cut the bodies to pieces. And not just because they were stoned, I don't think. It was something to do. It made a boring, depressing task more interesting. No one was really watching them. No one was supervising. It was really kind of gruesome in a sense. Autopsies are gruesome, anyway, but to have that kind of lack of regard for peoples' bodies . . . Of course, no one knew about this, because they'd put all that stuff back inside, and they'd be done. But I think it happened basically because there was no one sitting there, concerned about what might happen to those veterans. It was not as if they had families, many of them, to watch out for them. I don't think that could happen as easily in a community hospital because there would be relatives around who would act in the individual interest of the patient. But in the VA, there wasn't that. No one really cared."

Berliner, who also did a brief stint as an administrative resident at the Boston VA, is likewise critical of the arrangement whereby medical schools and VA hospitals are constructed in close proximity. "It's basically financial," he says, "and it's purely for the medical school."

Noting the high incidence of heart surgery at the Harvard-affiliated West Roxbury VA at the time, Berliner suggests that "in some way it was a consulting racket, because the VA had very high consulting fees. It may have been that these were very fine consultants, and the level of care was high, but one never got the sense of that being around there.

"My sense was that this was a place that gave the medical school a certain amount of extra clinical material, a very free rein in terms of operating, a very free rein in terms of increasing their own power. It used to be said that the Deans' Committee ran the hospital, and I think that was for the most part true. And as such it really did become just an adjunct to the medical school. It was a toy or a tool."

Berliner adds that the ease with which medical schools were able to get the VA to purchase fancy equipment that the school, by itself, could not afford enhanced the VA's self-image as a teaching institution.

"Essentially, it sets up the veteran as a guinea pig. Not just because of oversurgery, but because if they had the equipment, they felt they had to use it. In the VA, who is going to protest doing operating? It was a good place to get experience. It was a limited experience, only elderly men for the most part, but getting the technique was what counted.

"I suspect there were a lot of things that went on that were medically unjustifiable, in a strict sense. But at least you were getting some attention. Doctors spoke to you more than they usually did, for example. But I don't have a real sense that the VA is a really appropriate way to give medical care. Obviously, you have to learn on somebody. And it was a good way for the VA to get good physicians, with academic appointments. But it gave up a lot. It gave up patient care as a first priority. That's not a very good way for a hospital to operate."

Residents were doing other unsupervised things in the early seventies, which neither the VA nor the medical school nor the ubiquitous Deans' Committee knew anything about. If they did, they would probably have been more upset than any amount of publicity about too much heart surgery or stoned autopsies could have generated. Yet, in this case, the doctors, caught up in the idealism of the times, if not of their profession, were saving lives —without affiliation approval or knowledge.

For at least two years, 1970–72, a draft-evasion ring was run out of the medical research laboratories at the Boston VA hospital. It was well organized and popular.

"It could only have been done in a VA hospital," says someone with firsthand knowledge of the operation's existence, "because, typically, no one had any control or idea of what was going on anywhere in the place, not just in the research labs.

"Basically, a group of radical doctors would give medical examinations to draft-eligible men, find something wrong with them, and write medical letters for their medical deferment."

It was the height of antiwar activity throughout the country, and the doctors, in violation of VA policy, were, ironically, seeing "patients" *before* they became veterans in order to prevent them from showing up, disabled, after they had already become veterans. It was a heady time, and their good offices were sought out eagerly.

"The administration of the hospital knew nothing about this, again because in any other hospital if you gave somebody a blood test, somebody would have to pay for it," explains the observer, himself in frequent, close contact with hospital administrators during that period. "In the VA, no one had to pay for it. Things were marked 'research' for 'Dr. So-and-so' and no one ever questions it. The lab didn't question it. They just looked at volume. They didn't look at who was getting what.

"The [participating] doctors would give them chemical tests to try and find deficiencies in something, or give people drugs and then do the testing and definitely find something.

"All these facilities were being used for draft evasion in the veterans' hospital. No one at the hospital knew they were being treated. They walked in the front door, and went up to the doctors' offices and dealt with individual doctors, not as part of the VA, but just using these facilities. It was free blood testing, free laboratory testing. Some of the doctors involved were research staff, some were residents.

"People found out about it through a very informal kind of word of mouth. I had a friend who told other friends at college. Some people he met for lunch in the hospital cafeteria after his test."

At the time of the draft-evasion program, the hospital administration was busy defending its action permitting the sale of anti-war newspapers in the hospital lobby. Bitterly opposed by the major service organizations, the permission was granted as part of the hospital's efforts to appear more sympathetic to the younger veteran. One result was that it was more preoccupied than usual with concerns other than those that were related directly to the running of the hospital.

"While all that was going on downstairs," the observer adds, "people were being given draft-evasion physicals upstairs. It must have been an unusual sight to see a lot of young men floating around who didn't look like veterans."

Thanks to the VA, the U.S. military lost the services of several hundred draft-age recruits. And, in return, the VA had removed from it the potential burdens of providing beds and care for those Selective Service evaders who might otherwise have gone to Vietnam and returned wounded and in need of medical benefits.

A rare example, indeed, of the VA, resident doctors, and "patients" sharing the fruits of affiliation.

But the issues are not restricted to the lapses in supervision at selected VA hospitals, or to the abusive treatment of individual veterans. They are much more far-reaching than that, touching on the very role of American medicine itself, and its breeding grounds, the American medical school. The American Medical Association, for example, has never been happy with the VA system, raising as it does (for some) the specter of socialized medicine.

(For others it does the opposite. "It's enough to make me a Republican," says one critic of the VA who considers himself a socialist. "If that's socialized medicine, then I'm all for tripling the medical fees of veterans.")

Originally conceived to help returning World War II doctors finish their training as well as alleviate a health manpower shortage, medical training in VA hospitals under the auspices of affiliated medical schools has outpaced initial intentions. Dale M. Swayngim, VFW state service officer for North Carolina, put it clearly in his statement to the House medical facilities and benefits subcommittee when he said that "the original planners, I believe, foresaw interns and residents pursuing a career through the Veterans Administration. This has not happened, as this [medical school] dominance assures fidelity to their parent institution, not to the Veterans Administration.

"Thus, we have a medical school influence with patient services provided by the intern and the resident whose loyalty and short tenure is programmed to the parent institution and to his self-interest, not to the total Veterans Administration."

Berliner suggests this attitude may be different in a private hospital "where the physicians have, in a sense, a pecuniary interest in the patients. It's not just that you operate once and you never see them again. It's that you want to see them again, you want them to come back to you or tell their friends about you. That's not the case in the VA. So you lose that incentive. It may be a bad incentive, but it's one of the few things going for the system that makes it work correctly."

Add to that the relatively low salary levels for VA physicians —in 1975, VA doctors earned two-thirds the salaries of Defense Department and Public Health Service doctors, even less when certain fringe benefits are added into the military employees' pot.

Until recently, the most a VA physician could earn was slightly more than $55,000 a year, still several thousand dollars under the *average* DOD and PHS levels. In August 1980 Congress voted overwhelmingly, over a presidential veto, to increase the pay to as much as $76,200.

In addition, a recent survey shows that almost 60 percent of the physicians who resign each year from the VA would have stayed if VA compensation "had approximated that offered other federal physicians." Further, 82 percent of those resigning were specialty-board certified. Among certain specialties, vacancy rates are extremely high at the VA: 77 percent in neurology, 55 percent in anesthesiology, and 37 percent in radiology.

Currently, concludes the June 24, 1977, report by the private consultant firm Coopers and Lybrand, "the VA is unable to recruit young, well-trained, full-time physicians into the medical system." In short, the government provides for its own when its own —read: active-duty servicemen and -women—are in uniform. But once the khaki is shed, the quality and quantity of the health-care providers are no longer touted—or assured.

The VA is suffering a severe shortage of full-time physicians. As late as 1979, thirty-two VA hospitals had a majority of doctors working part time, including one hospital, Birmingham, where an incredible 91.6 percent were on part-time status. In seven hospitals, the chief of staff, the most important doctor at the facility, is a part-timer. In most cases, the part-time VA chief of staff is also employed by the medical school. According to VA regulations as well as common VA practice, these part-timers can be removed at the recommendation of the school, in effect giving the university virtually complete control over the chief of staff position— and the medical functioning of the hospital.

Further weakening the VA's position are the results of a National Research Council study that revealed that most part-time VA doctors place their allegiance outside of the VA system. "If the present trend continues," worried Florida Senator Richard Stone, "I fear that nearly all of our VA facilities will have to rely upon medical specialists and general practitioners who can provide only a fraction of their time to the medical needs of our veterans."

The 1978 VA annual report informs that, via its health-care education and training efforts, "developing sufficient numbers of all categories of professional and other health personnel to help meet the needs of the VA" is *secondary* to educating and training health-care professionals who, having utilized the VA as a training ground, generally seek full-time employment outside of the VA system. It is estimated, for example, that well over 50 percent of physicians practicing in the United States today have had some medical training at a VA facility. But the number of those staying on to work at the VA is infinitesimal, leaving the VA—and the veteran on whom the learning was done—without the benefit of the finished product of the training arrangement.

Some say one way to overcome this deficit may be to make training opportunities contingent on the trainee's agreement, in writing, to "pay back" his or her use of veterans for learning purposes, by spending a specified period of time at a VA facility. Both the military and the Public Health Service have arrangements like this, and the National Health Service, where newly minted doctors work in underserved rural or inner city areas, is expanding its program into selected urban hospitals and prisons.

Designating VA hospitals as underserved would solve two immediate problems: It would make the public aware of the low-priority status accorded veterans, and it would relieve some of the pressures brought about by a chronic doctor shortage.

But don't count on it.

Says the assistant dean of a small medical school, himself sympathetic to the plight of the underserved rural population of his state, "Just try and get residents to pay back at the VA. They'll tell you to stick it in your ear. No one wants to work at the VA if they can help it."

Sometimes they can't help it.

In the early 1960s, as a young psychology trainee, I spent three months at the Gulfport VA hospital on the Mississippi Gulf Coast. It is a large psychiatric "station," as it was then called, set among the palms across U.S. 90 from a segregated beach. This was the summer before James Meredith was to change the course of history at the University of Mississippi.

My room on the second floor of the staff dormitory was adequate enough, equipped as it was with the South's most important piece of machinery—a working fan. The room was no more than fifteen feet from an active east-west freight line, and the first morning the 4:39 came roaring by, I knew for sure my trembling cot was about to be reduced to roadbed.

That turned out to be the least of my worries.

A few weeks after I arrived in early June, I was joined by a half-dozen medical students from Ole Miss, there to spend a summer's clerkship. The assortment of future doctors the VA was about to help train was fascinating—and frightening.

I remember several of the students vividly. (Their identities have been changed here.)

Frankie—the most personable, who spoke with the clarity of a man underwater with delta mud in his mouth, and who frequently bragged about how many courses he still had to make up because of failing grades, and who, on our nightly sojourns to the local bars along the technically dry strip—where liquor was sold illegally and openly—would never forget to remind the raucous mixture of truck mechanics, farmers, and other native folk that I was a "nigger-lover from New York."

George—now a practicing physician in Knoxville, whose federal judge uncle was making national headlines busily handing down antidesegregation rulings, and who was the most fair-minded of the bunch, owing he said, to the fact that he had served in the air force and, therefore, had rid himself of that blasted provincialism, and who would, responding to periodic marital problems, guiltily wander off to a well-known woman who, he said, pleaded with him to "tear up my pussy, please."

John—continually drunk because, he said, all the men in his family had died by age thirty, and since he had only a few more years to go, it didn't bother him much to show up besotted at medical rounds and other assigned hospital chores and, anyway, most of the patients were "crazy niggers."

Tom—who everyone cheerfully agreed would wind up with a large female clientele because he had a way with women, and who talked of his joy in tying off the tubes, unrequested and unannounced, of nigger women down at the county hospital in Jackson so they couldn't have no more nigger babies.

Pete—the most vicious of all, from Pelham Parkway in the Bronx, who was drunk most of the time, too, excusing it, when he was sober, by his tough childhood and by the fact that this summer, after all, was the last period of freedom for him and his buddies, since they would soon have to go out and earn a living.

Several weeks after they settled in, we were told that the chief of psychology from the Tuscaloosa VA would be staying at the dorm for the weekend. When the medical students found out the forthcoming visitor was black, they went berserk.

It's hard now, almost twenty years later, to recall the utter disbelief and then fear that I experienced as these future health-care professionals went screaming through the halls demanding he be given a separate toilet, separate drinking fountain, separate stairway, separate floor, separate dining quarters, separate life. . . .

I thought they were joking, the display was so outlandish and irrational. My tentative amusement, however, turned to distress when I asked George, the worldly-wise air force man, how serious they were. "They might kill him if he shows up," George said matter-of-factly.

They didn't, of course, but my offer to eat supper with the man —whose terrified reaction to my knock on his door is something, even after twenty years, I haven't forgotten—resulted in the end of my relationship with the medical students. That night, as I lay in my bed listening to the continued ranting of the group—now drunkenly angry beyond reason because a man with a Ph.D. whose skin was black was living temporarily within pissing distance—Frankie threatened to break my door down (as near as I could understand him) and show me some real southern hospitality.

The whoosh-whoosh of the fan finally soothed me to sleep, and I awoke the following morning to the glares of the other whites on the floor.

Although they knew about the incident, no one in authority at the hospital ever spoke to the students involved. It also bothered nobody that a Dr. Rodriguez, a personable psychiatrist from South America, couldn't communicate with his patients because he didn't speak English too well. I remember all of us, including the Mississippi medical students, chuckling over that one.

The original legislation creating the Department of Medicine and Surgery back in 1946 also allowed for the establishment of a medical residency program whereby individuals with M.D. degrees and at least one year of postgraduate training could continue their education at VA facilities and at the government's expense. However, not only were residents being trained, but even in the absence of specific authorization, so were interns (less advanced medical school graduates—"unskilled personnel," the VA now calls them) and medical students, the very people previous administrators swore would not be allowed in to practice on "guinea pig" veterans.

Replying to Congressman Rankin's stated worry at congressional hearings that letting the medical schools into the VA hospitals would result in "inexperienced doctors" working on "guinea pig" patients, General Bradley, testifying in support of the proposed DM&S in 1945, said that the residents "are not people that are still studying medicine. . . . They have finished their internship." The statement is a clear rejection of the use of medical students or interns in the new setup.

Quick to take advantage, however, of the VA's sloppy, unmonitored, and essentially passive attitude—as long as the medical schools wanted in it was okay with the VA—the schools soon began violating the original agreement, although they temporized. Their position is summarized in this 1949 quote by the man serving as chief of medical services at the Louisville VA and as associate professor of medicine at the affiliated University of Louisville School of Medicine. He wrote in the *Southern Medical Journal:*

It soon became evident that there was a wealth of *teaching material* in the hospital, and inasmuch as nearly all of the full-time staff and all of the consultant staff were already members of the faculty of the University of Louisville School of Medicine, it was felt desirable that *medical students* of the University be rotated through the hospital for teaching purposes. Accordingly, senior medical students were assigned to the hospital in July, 1946 . . . [Italics added.]

In 1948, the VA specifically allowed, still without legal authority and contrary to the explicit wishes of Congress and the promises of General Bradley, medical students to be appointed "clinical clerks without compensation." Benjamin Lewis reports that Congress continued to be uneasy with the VA's use of medical students. The discontent, he notes, "was related to the possible harmful effect on veterans' care." He cites the 1947 House Special Committee: "they [the VA] should see to it that the hospital does not become a training ground for medical students rather than a veterans' hospital with the veterans receiving proper treatment."

In an attempt to remove some of the stigma of illegality and irresponsibility, the VA got Congress to include specifically the training of interns within the affiliation structure. On September 2, 1958, along with codification of the laws administered by the VA, interns finally were permitted to train, legally, in the VA, although they had been treating patients there for more than ten years already.

In 1973, still showing some uncertainty, the VA elaborated on the duties and responsibilities of interns (and residents) after veterans' groups and others continued to question the legal status of some of those providing care for their comrades. And in 1976, thirty years after interns first entered VA hospitals and eighteen years after they were first legally permitted in them, the VA went out of its way to define who an intern was.

In none of this was the status of the medical student brought up.

According to Guy McMichael III, the VA's general counsel, the authority for using medical students at VA facilities is in Title 38 of the U.S. Code. He points to this wording: "The Administrator . . . may employ . . . physicians, dentists . . . and other . . . unskilled personnel (including interns, residents, trainees, and students in medical support programs)." Traditionally, however, "medical support" programs refer to nursing, psychology, and other nonmedical but medically related disciplines. Medical students are students in medicine, not supportive of it. The fact that their VA title is "clinical clerk" and they work at the VA in "clinical clerk-ships" belies the contention they are allowed within the VA hospital under Title 38 auspices—or any other auspice.

Additionally, since Congress, previous VA administrators, and veterans themselves have historically strongly rejected the inclusion of medical students in the VA training programs, it would appear that only *specific,* clear-cut authorizing legislation would allow them on the wards. The precedent for that has been established—for residents in 1946 and, after enough outcry, for interns in 1958. There is no similar legislation for medical students, and veterans' complaints of being treated by unqualified personnel may, after all these years, still be legitimate.

At least one person knowledgeable about the whole affiliation arrangement suggests that the role of the medical student is related to the relative power balance between the two institutions involved. "Generally in some medical-school-dominated relationships, there is probably too much unsupervised or inadequately supervised authority allowed to be exercised by medical students, particularly in admitting areas," says Jonathan Steinberg, chief counsel to Senator Alan Cranston's Committee on Veterans' Affairs.

Steinberg, who emphasizes that he is speaking only for himself personally, also says the affiliation is a worthwhile endeavor. He calls it "a highly valuable, probably indispensable (for both the VA and the school) relationship." Although the relative influence fluctuates, he adds that "right now more medical schools are more dominant . . . than five, ten years ago and than VA medical centers are."

Noting that the committee may legislatively address "any perceived imbalance," he says, "Certainly, there are instances where the reality of operations is not what the policy or regulations call for." He doubts, however, that there is a basis for "serious challenge to the statutory authority of the VA . . . regarding affiliations and medical students."

Steinberg's, and McMichael's, arguments fly in the face of impassioned statements like those of Dr. Paul Schafer, Oliver Meadows and others who take it for granted that the VA is quite vulnerable legally. In fact, the historical attitudes of both Congress and previous VA administrators like Bradley, not to mention Steinberg's characterization of serious lapses in the entire affiliation/medical student relationship, raise critical questions about the program's future. Indeed, the situation may just be waiting for some enterprising public law firm (and an angry veteran) to come along and take the matter to court.

"It was deemed necessary to add specific authorizing legislation for interns," says Michael Browde, a professor of administrative law at the University of New Mexico School of Law and an expert in the field. "This would give rise to a strong inference that use of students is not sanctioned by Congress. Given the history of the development of the legislation, anything less than full doctors [i.e., anyone with no M.D. degree] requires specific legislation. There is a colorable [that is, legally arguable] claim there."

The question of medical student involvement in patient care is a serious one, because with staff shortages and other cutbacks, hospitals are relying more and more on nonphysician personnel, medical students among them. When a veteran enters a VA hospital, or any hospital, he expects to be treated by the most qualified people available. This isn't necessarily the case.

A veteran from Oregon writes in *Stars and Stripes,* "I was cared for by medical students. You are right about getting medical students out of VA hospitals. Let them practice on nonveterans. When will VA change their policy and practices and make supervision for medical students mandatory?" A full-time VA doctor, fed up with deteriorating care in the system, wrote about medical records he has seen: "All treatment was by a third-year medical student. When it was felt that a consultation was indicated, it was done by a fourth-year medical student."

A second-year medical student, just finishing his clerkship in internal medicine at a medium-sized VA hospital, says, "We did all the work there. I hardly knew what I was doing. All the doctors were too busy to supervise us, or they forgot about us. Fortunately, I didn't have to see too many patients who were seriously ill. If I did, well . . . I'm just glad I didn't."

The problems of supervision are not confined to those with pre-M.D. status. Responding to charges in April 1979 from an anonymous caller that residents' unsupervised surgery at the Manhattan VA caused some patients to die, Carl A. Sensi of the VA's Inspector General's office concluded that the chief of the surgical service, Dr. Alex C. Solowey, a professor at the NYU School of Medicine, "did not adequately supervise that service."

Included in the substantiated charges was the fact that the attending M.D.s' notes, required to document all surgical and other medical procedures, "were often prepared and signed by residents—sometimes without the knowledge and approval of the attending physician. . . . These were not isolated incidents." In other words, the notes, which if properly signed would indicate the mandated presence of appropriate, immediately available supervision by an experienced surgeon, were forged.

Against all rules and propriety, some residents even performed surgery when their supervisors were on leave, affixing signatures to make it appear as if they were present in or around the operating room. The inspector general, deciding that patient care did not suffer and no deaths occurred from these written and supervisory lapses involving "inadequate and incomplete" notes, recommended that a professional standards board review the performance of Dr. Solowey, that the criteria for obtaining patient consent be clarified and standardized (already done years earlier), and that medical record-keeping deficiencies at the medical center be corrected.

"What I object to," says Rep. Lester Wolff, the former New York Congress member who demanded an investigation, "is the lack of supervision of doctors in training. They require supervision."

Somehow, inadequate record-keeping doesn't affect the quality of medical care, according to the VA. That makes it hard to understand, of course, why there should be any records, or supervision, at all—until one remembers the influence of the medical school.

Beyond that is the tension inherent in serving two, ostensibly equal, masters: The resident gets paid by the VA, but supervised, trained, and evaluated by the medical school.

"It is quite clear that the supervision of the residents lies with the medical school," says Tom Sherwood, the Manhattan VA administrator whose NYU-affiliated hospital was the subject of the inspector general's report. "But the chief of services, also on the faculty of the school, is supposed to be responsible for the physicians in that he dictates to some degree their education as a function of the patient's needs for the particular service that he's providing. I can tell you there are tremendous conflicts in certain circumstances where that does not work."

Sherwood points out that resident assignments scheduled by a chief of service, based presumably on patient needs, may be ignored by the medical school. Sometimes, he says, some wards go uncovered as a result. "If it meets the goals of the medical school in terms of what they are doing for their program, then it will take precedence. From my experience, the medical school tends to dominate. The question is, then, if that is so, how are they able to effect the domination?

"Well, clearly, if they are paying the chief of surgery an additional sixteen thousand dollars over his salary, this is, I think, a very effective means. Don't forget, it's not just the sixteen thousand that counts to physicians. His appointment is also terribly important. The idea of being a full or an associate professor on a prestigious roster of the medical school is extremely important to him. And there is no telling, therefore, what kinds of arrangements he must make to protect that."

"The university basically has a different mandate," explains Dr. Herbert Rose, associate chief of staff for Research and Development at the Bronx Kingsbridge VA Medical Center and Paul Schafer's predecessor as president of the National Association of VA Physicians. He has been with the VA since 1962.

"But as part of the affiliation agreement, which gives them responsibility only for education, they control staffing, which has a tremendous impact on patient care. Essentially, they can determine the quality of patient care, and they have so much other power, the Deans' Committee, that they can have an enormous impact throughout the hospital. That was the intention of the program in the first place.

"But it creates some conflict regarding the interests of the vet-

eran. The veteran wants to get into the hospital because he feels
he's entitled, he's a sick veteran, he's entitled under the law. The
university, on the other hand, wants to admit people because it's
a teaching hospital. And young doctors have a tremendous
amount of power in university hospitals today. They can march
on the hospital and pee in the wastebasket of the chief of medicine if he doesn't do what they want. Or they quit.

"So they want to admit patients of interest for teaching purposes. There's an inherent conflict. It's hard to balance the patient's need, which should be the deciding factor, against these
kinds of pressures," Rose says. "It creates problems."

Rose adds that the conflict is not unique to the VA. It's true of
any teaching hospital, he says. Except, of course, that in VA hospitals, the medical schools have available to them all the patients,
an advantage which even the university's own (private) teaching
hospitals don't necessarily have.

In those latter facilities, traditionally only the patients catego-
rized as medically indigent have been freely used as teaching
material.

One of the people whose job is to grapple with those problems
is Dr. Paul East, the VA's bright and very thoughtful chief, Medical-Dental Division, in the central office's Education Service. East
was the sharpest and most insightful VA official I met in Washington. In fact, his outspoken, coherent views may have prompted
his exit from a similar position at HEW.

He has an M.D. in preventive medicine and also holds a law
degree.

"I've never been a patient in a hospital," he says, "so this is
total personal conjecture. But I would guess that most patients
who are weak [from their illness] probably don't want to be bothered too much by people in the hospital. The majority of others
probably don't mind as much being examined by a lot of different
people. The teaching situation, though, is not able to selectively
use hale and hearty patients, and no one else.

"Historically, medicine gives lip service in that regard, that
patients by selection, quote-unquote, are bargaining for multiple
examination exposure. Outside of the hospital setting, all those

examinations would be degrading. In the hospital, it depends on how it's handled for, it to be degrading or not. However, from a societal point of view, you can make the general statement: Without patients there can be no learning."

But East, who is from England, acknowledges the baggage involved.

"Patients who go to a teaching hospital bear the burden of that; those who don't, don't have that burden. There's no question that VA hospitals that have affiliations are better. All are better for it. They recruit better people, good people. Care is better because the people who are giving the care are better. Without the affiliations, quality would suffer."

East does exhibit some doubts about the whole process, however.

"I'm sure there could be fewer people doing the examinations and more use of audiovisual aids for training purposes on the wards. By and large, the [affiliated] setting will be better for the patient than not. But," he admits, "the patient has little choice."

There are those who argue that it's the physician, not the patient, whose choice is limited. Dr. Kiser, on the faculty of Texas' Southwestern School of Medicine in Dallas, would like to see more freedom given to the local levels. "The VA needs to realize that for any service to be of high quality it must be associated with a medical school and have facilities for research and training. They go hand in hand with good patient care."

They also go hand in glove with substantial benefits to the medical schools, at taxpayer expense.

By affiliating with the VA, for example, medical schools do not have to spend millions of dollars for medical and nursing supplies, advanced medical equipment, hospital beds, facility upkeep and maintenance, and, of course, teaching staff. Additionally, the VA pays for, and the medical schools use, consulting, attending, and part-time physicians. Basically, this is a lucrative mechanism whereby medical school faculty may supplement their income on a continuous, recurring schedule.

The amounts of money involved can be enormous.

For instance, in 1975 the VA spent $10 million to pay for non-VA "contracted" radiologists, anesthesiologists, and pathologists. More than $4 million of this money was paid to the university employers of these physicians for indirect or overhead expenses. The scenario is repeated annually.

In the same year at the West Haven, Connecticut, VA hospital, a radiology service contract was negotiated with the affiliated Yale University Medical School. As reported by the unofficial newspaper of American veterans, *Stars and Stripes,* the total cost was $255,382, of which $176,125 was for the base salary of the doctors. However, "The VA was required to pay the University $47,554 in 'fringe benefits' plus $31,703 in 'overhead.'

"Thus," the paper points out, "the University received $79,257 *more* than the salaries for that year, or 45 percent more than the VA would pay to its own VA physicians"—and overhead has risen to 85 percent at some schools since then.

Other publicity-shy benefits lavished on the medical schools include virtually free use of VA land and facilities for training purposes (over $1.1 billion worth of replacement medical centers, plant modernization, and research facility construction in 1978 alone), VA assumption of residents' and interns' salaries, unrestricted use of certain expensive lab equipment (VA-financed medical and prosthetic research topped $117 million in 1978), input into the design of new VA hospitals so that the schools' interests—teaching and research—might be better served (at an estimated 1978 construction cost for research and education projects of $25.2 million), payment by the VA of the indirect costs (food, supplies, staff) of allowing medical students on the wards, and de facto financial control of millions of dollars in staff salaries.

Not a bad arrangement for institutions with no direct public accountability.

It is precisely this kind of setup, consumer critics assert, that encourages a *decrease* in medical attention to veterans, while fostering an increase in the prestige and power of the education moguls. "The doctors spend all their time with their students, and very little time with the patients," charges a service organization representative at the Fresno, California, VA Medical Center. On the wall in his small office, one of four in a row serving as quarters for veterans' organizations on the hospital's ground floor, is a red and white bumper sticker: "Hire the vet—Veterans make good employees."

The 265-bed facility, first opened in 1947, has been affiliated with the University of California, San Francisco, for four years. Because of its size—it is small for a VA facility—it appears to be more like a local community hospital than part of a nationwide chain.

Though a little shoddy around the edges, it is clean and well kept, except in those areas where remodeling at the medical school's request has disrupted the peace and tranquillity patients had come to expect. It projects a friendly, easygoing atmosphere —much like the director who runs it.

"Starting an affiliation is a very traumatic process," acknowledges Wallace R. Koseluk, with the VA thirty-two years, including two tours at the central office, and Fresno's administrator the past three and a half. "But in the end, it's very clear it improves patient care." He echoes the sentiments of other hospital directors, like Durham's B. Fred Brown, who talk of the transition tensions an affiliation provokes.

"Physicians weren't interested in coming here," he says. "Now, with the university, we're gradually getting more doctors. It's a very emotional issue. If you say patient care is better with the affiliation, you run into criticism that the physicians here before were incompetent, insensitive, unqualified, et cetera. That's obviously not true. Now we have some real heavies in terms of qualifications. We have specialties we never had before: ophthalmology, gastroenterology.

"One of the big problems is the change in the method of delivery of care. In an affiliated institution, whether it's the VA or a private or community hospital, care is not provided in the same way. Residents give bedside care, but a lot of teaching goes on.

"There is an impact on the veteran who's been coming here the last ten years and been used to more hand-holding personal care, perhaps, although physicians coming out of medical school now are aware of the need to personalize care, though it's different. There are staff who don't fit into the new kind of care, physicians who are generalists, and find it hard to function as a teacher-specialist. It's a half-fish, half-fowl organization. It takes many years to evolve an organization like an affiliated organization.

"All of the efforts suddenly begin to jell. We've gone from utter poverty in positions to many house staff. One problem is that the resources don't keep up with the growth. It's hell getting enough technicians, nurses, and operating funds to support the higher-level care. The system is very slow to accommodate that kind of change."

Nor is the system—that is, the VA and the medical schools—quick to point that out, to make it a visible part of its public balance sheet. On one side of the ledger are the hidden benefits accruing to the medical schools. On the other side are the crushing costs to the VA, in harried, overworked staff and lessening patient care.

While the Veterans Administration crows about the positive impact that affiliations have on patient care, it conveniently ignores, and Congress overlooks, the stark fact that without increases in staff to support the influx of all these young, talented doctors and their high-paid experienced specialist teachers—without more nurses, more clerks, more assistants, more *help*—the patient's gain is nothing more than an allegation spent in the coin of a medical school's prestige.

The charade is nationwide, and far from recent.

"The continuous growth of the [University of New Mexico] medical school affiliation has not been met with a corresponding growth in hospital staff, especially at the support level," Paul Schmoll, former Albuquerque VA hospital director, reported to the House Committee on Veterans' Affairs in 1974. "This has resulted in an increased burden of work on the personnel involved in direct patient care and ancillary staff."

In other words, the veteran is getting stuck with less quality care, not more, as advertised—despite the mighty med school's arrival on the scene. Not surprisingly, then, consumers like the Fresno service officer who spent twenty-one years in the air force, are not sure the change is worth it. "Although there's now a surplus of physicians [at the hospital]," he says, "they're not enough to satisfy the needs of the patients we have." A patient is seen within twenty-four hours, he claims, but infrequently thereafter. Further, a patient may be seen by a doctor only two or three times during a ten-day stretch.

But there's more.

"Patients complain they're used as guinea pigs," he relates, raising a not unfamiliar refrain. "If a patient has a rare abnormality, he's swarmed over by physician-instructors and students. He's prodded, poked, and everything else. It has to be something of academic interest for the students. The hospital staff hasn't taken kindly to that.

"The VA system is very much needed in the overall picture of things. I don't want to make it sound all bad. The VA is vitally important. It takes a terrific burden off the other hospitals in the area. By and large it does a good job with the facilities they have. But it has internal problems which need to be solved."

"No one wants the medical school out," agrees Reason Warehime, a World War II and Korean War army veteran who spends a lot of time at the hospital. "We just want the system to work with what we have."

Director Koseluk insists it does.

"In some ways we get the best of everything and sort of escape the worst of it" is the way he assesses the matter. "I don't feel the least bit dominated by the university. Personalities have a lot to do with it. If we have any problems, we're almost like brothers under the skin. We put our heads together to do what we both feel has to be done.

"I can't recall any real disagreement."

In 1978, by way of punctuation, the VA agreed to build a $1.2-million Area Health Education Center at Fresno for use by the University of California–San Francisco Medical School.

"It'll be a nice addition," says Koseluk.

But when millions of dollars are at stake, and perhaps your job, it is easy to rationalize away the criticism.

"I would say there is no hospital in this country where you couldn't elicit complaints," declares Dr. Leonard Napolitano with a full measure of certainty.

Napolitano, wound up and solemn, his skin the color of tobacco, is the dean of the University of New Mexico School of Medicine, affiliated with the Albuquerque VA Medical Center.

"People are frightened and anxious when they enter a hospital. Hospitals are frightening places for people."

Asserting that "doctors are human, too, they need sleep like anyone else," he adds, "There are a lot of drunks, a lot of men out there [at the VA] who can be extremely irritating."

Napolitano, a Ph.D. in anatomy, is something of a rarity. He is only one of a small handful of medical school deans who do not have a medical degree (M.D.). Still, his attitude is important, especially so because it is reflected in the product turned out by the fifteen-year-old school.

For Paul [a pseudonymous second-year medical student at UNM whose story was told in the Albuquerque *Journal*], perhaps the most frustrating and discouraging thing about his internal medicine rotation was the setting in which it occurred—the [Albuquerque] VA hospital.

The building was old and without air-conditioning. Administration was typically bureaucratic. Decisions to admit patients were related to the "average daily patient load" since funding for the hospital was calculated on that basis.

Worst of all, the patients were ones who made it very difficult for Paul to be the way he preferred to be— compassionate, empathetic and caring. They were frequently elderly men, alcoholics, or uncontrolled diabetics who smoked too much, didn't like longhaired young doctors, and acted as if they thought the world owed them everything.

Paul felt a conflict in relating to these kinds of patients, believing on the one hand that everyone had a right to health care, yet condemning their self-destructive lifestyles and failure to contribute to society.

It takes no great leap of imagination to understand that Paul, like his medical student and resident counterparts elsewhere, is reacting to what he has learned from his elders—from the dean on down. A medical school setting that emphasized compassion and empathy—along with skills in taking blood pressure and making accurate diagnoses—would not graduate students who flinch from the prospects of ministering to supposedly difficult patients.

It is easy to forget that no one is forced to enter the practice of medicine.

There should be no compelling reasons, then, why the Pauls of our medical schools cannot be prepared by their distinguished mentors to respond with equanimity, sensitivity, and assurance to the hurts of those who supposedly may be remiss in their contributions to society.

The welfare-mentality shuck clothed in hospital white.

Paul, no doubt, is also unaware of the tenuous legal status of the medical student on the VA ward, or the historical concerns of veterans and veterans' groups that the medical schools would replace the patient's treatment goals with their primary interest in teaching fledgling doctors—like Paul.

They didn't teach him that, either, in medical school.

It is, in all, a telling commentary.

The purpose of medical research is not to work on the birds and bees. The purpose is to make lives more comfortable.

— *Dr. Rosalyn Yalow, VA researcher and 1977 Nobel Prize winner*

4

SIGNING UP TO DIE

When it needs help, the VA can always work with the military to create problems for the veterans—life-threatening problems. Peter Watson swears to it.

AFFIDAVIT

I, Peter Watson, of Los Angeles, California, depose and say:

1. Having been in the military service I was eligible for VA treatment. In early 1967 I read about the Water Program at Wadsworth Veterans Hospital. This was a weight-loss program and because I was obese I went there and spoke to [Dr. K.] about getting on the program. In March 1967 I was told that I might be a candidate for the program. It was my understanding that on this program I would be taking water and would lose weight from malnutrition.

2. Before beginning the program, I was given a psychiatric and medical examination. The medical examination included a liver biopsy. I was not told of the results of the examination at the time I entered into the program. I later learned through my malpractice suit in 1977 that the liver biopsy had indicated that I had a bad liver previous to beginning

116

the program. I should not have been accepted to the Water Program because of my liver condition.

I was given a consent form to sign. At the time I signed the consent form I was under the influence of Stelazine, Thorazine, Melaril, and Dilantin. I did not read the form but I did sign it. I didn't receive a copy of it.

It was the opinion of others in the program that the consent form was for the liver biopsy. This was what I thought to be true. The only benefit I was told I would get from the program was loss of weight. I was not warned of any possible side effects or risks from the program.

3. There were forty other persons in the program and we were divided up in groups of three. Three times a day I was given Dilantin and one other drug which was supposed to counteract gout. Other than those medications I was only given water. There was no other form of nutrition.

I was not told before the start of the program that I would be taking the medications. Previous to the program I had been taking Dilantin for a military injury to the central nervous system. The purpose of taking the drug was to arrest seizures that I had from the military injury.

During the water Program [Dr. K.] kept me on Dilantin. I would spend my days at the hospital lying in bed or walking around. They would regularly take urine samples and give me blood tests. They would also check my lungs.

About two weeks into the starvation diet I started having seizures. I asked the doctor why I was still having seizures as I had been taking Dilantin which was supposed to prevent them. He did not answer my question. The seizures would cause me to fall down or pass out.

The program lasted for forty-eight days and much of that time I was depressed. I got more and more depressed as time went on. Towards the end of the program I had a complete nervous breakdown. I was lying on my bed and crying. I wasn't sure of the reason for my depression but when I had the breakdown I was taken off the program and sent to Ward I28A of the Psychiatric Division of Brentwood [VA] Hospital.

I was at the hospital for three days, at which time my wife signed me out. [Dr. K.] had told me that when I quieted down he wanted me to get right back on the program, but after I was released from Brentwood Hospital they would not let me back on the program. I was not told the reason for this and I was given no medical follow-up from Wadsworth VA.

4. Since the program I have been involved in investigating the program and am currently involved in a malpractice suit. I have documents to prove that I had a liver condition before entering the program and that the program caused my liver to fail.

In 1977 the VA gave me an additional 30% service increase because of the determined damage to my liver caused by the narcotics. I also learned that the hospital report from Psychiatric Hospital stated that I was suffering from a toxic reaction to medication and they believed that that was the reason for my breakdown.

5. A few years later I learned from [Dr. K.] that the real purpose of the experiment was to determine the effects of starvation on the mind. This is why the air force was interested in the program. They had helped to finance it along with the Wadsworth VA, who supplied staff and housing. UCLA was also involved and [Dr. K.] also worked at UCLA [which is affiliated with Wadsworth].

[Dr. K.] told me that the purpose of the program was also to check malnutrition on the metabolic system and the reaction of Dilantin on the system without nutrition. There was an article in *Life* magazine a number of years back substantiating the financing of the program and other information concerning the Water Program.

6. As a result of taking the medications on the Water Program without any nutrition in my system my liver collapsed, which in turn has given me spleen and kidney problems. These problems are still with me today. I have to urinate up to twelve times a day and if I don't it is painful. I can't take any medication for my condition and I hope to get surgery.

I had no benefit from the program. I didn't lose weight. Had I known what I know now about the program I would never have entered into it.

I swear that the above statements are given of my own free will and volition. I also swear that the above statements are true and correct.

For Peter Watson (not his real name), obscured and cavalier experimentation have become sickening, fighting words. For others they will forever be whispers of a different kind.

In the balance books of the VA, Kenneth Chenin's life and death are measured by the weight of a tie vote. Nowhere is it recorded, however, whether Chenin, a forty-four-year-old Korean War–era veteran under treatment for hypertension, appreciated the irony of having his fate memorialized by the democratic principles he was so ceremoniously drafted to defend. Nonetheless, some contend, there is an increasingly voluminous ledger that strongly suggests that the VA, under whose benevolent auspices at Long Beach, California, this particular balloting transpired, makes decidedly casual use of those cherished American procedures.

Chenin himself took no part in the voting.

He was dead by the time the franchise was exercised. Indeed, there is evidence that he wasn't even told his life was being risked, when there still were alternatives open to him.

Chenin suffered a major cerebrovascular accident in September 1973, following a cardiac catheterization performed, apparently unknown to him or his family, for experimental research purposes at the Long Beach VA. No one at the hospital, including Dr. B., chief of the Cardiology Service and the study's principal investigator, bothered to tell him properly and in a timely manner about the experiment, "Therapy of hypertension with propranolol."

Neither did anyone request his written permission to involve him in the dangerous operation. In addition, as reported by Dr. Robert W. Porter, the hospital's associate chief of staff for Research and Development, in the August 27, 1973, minutes of the Human Studies Subcommittee,

Examination of the records in this case indicated that the patient [Chenin] had been placed on this study in April, 1973, *although the project was not approved until June 7, 1973.* Furthermore, *there was no informed consent* (Form 1086) *for the research study. . . .* It was further *noted that this patient did not meet the criteria set forth for the research proposal* which was subsequently approved on June 7. [Italics added.]

Nor were the "expected complications" accurately represented to the Research and Education Committee, one of the two committees whose approval was required for the study to proceed.

Porter's notes, the official minutes of the meeting, conclude with the statement that the subcommittee will recommend to the full Research and Education Committee, at its next gathering, that all cardiac catheterization for research purposes be halted.

At that meeting, in the hospital director's nicely appointed conference room, Dr. John R. Kent, chief of Endocrinology and chairperson of the Human Studies Subcommittee, reminded the eighteen committee members present of the "grave doubts" expressed at an earlier Research and Education meeting "regarding the propriety of left heart catheterization in patients in whom it was not otherwise clinically indicated."

Not far from where Kenneth Chenin's body once lay in the huge medical facility, Dr. Kent tells his distinguished colleagues, "The subcommittee is deeply concerned that the repetition of such occurrences at this hospital will ultimately lead to a severe restriction of all clinical research." Later, the committee will discuss the Nuremberg Code and the Declaration of Helsinki, which concerns itself with the rights of patients, as well as make reference to informed consent procedures issued by the California Medical Association (CMA).

With "risky diagnostic procedures," one doctor read from the CMA manual, "the physician has a duty to explain the nature of the procedure; any risks, regardless of their likelihood, which could cause serious bodily harm; and the alternative method of treatment, if any." The guidelines, which insistently underscore the right of the patient to be truly informed, further indicate that "it is essential that the physician personally discuss the matter with the patient and make detailed notes of the discussion and the patient's reactions in the patient's medical chart."

According to the committee's minutes, Dr. B. "responded that this patient had been treated on clinical [i.e., health care] grounds and that the research project had subsequently developed out of this clinical experience." He also stated that propranolol, the drug used as the focus of the experiment, was "fully approved and widely used in the treatment of hypertension and that, in his opinion, cardiac catheterization was clinically indicated for patients on this anti-hypertensive agent."

But B. did not mention, as his colleagues did, that, according to the minutes, "although propranolol is an approved drug in daily use, the FDA has approved its use only in cardiac arrhythmias [heartbeat irregularities] and its use in other areas must therefore be considered experimental. The discussion also emphasized that other modes of therapy which were less likely to produce adverse reactions are available and that patients should therefore be so informed."

B. outlined step-by-step precautions that would preclude in the future any criticism of his methods, indicating further that he felt the experimental procedure was not at fault in Chenin's case. B. then asked the committee for permission to complete his research.

Dr. Porter, who is presently chief of neurosurgery and temporary acting chief of surgery, sighs on a very hot late summer midday long after the Chenin-B. experiment has passed—September 6, 1979, exactly six years to the hour after Dr. B. held his *tête-à-tête* with the Research and Education Committee. Porter doesn't acknowledge the anniversary, but he does admit to some . . . problems, which he dismisses as procedural.

"It was a surgical consent, a consent for surgery, not research," he concedes, recalling the circumstances of Chenin's death. "Technically, it was a violation, but we did have the patient's consent for surgery. Still, we had the patient's consent, and we also had it verbally. We unwittingly used the wrong consent. Morally, the surgical consent was better than nothing."

Porter is not particularly perturbed, either, that Chenin was listed as participating in the research a full two months before the study got approval. "That's a technicality," he repeats. "He signed up early but nothing happened to the patient until the study was approved. The patient was recruited, so to speak, for the study but nothing was done to him [before it was okayed]."

Nor is Porter overly upset that, since Chenin didn't sign a research consent form, he obviously couldn't have agreed that he understood all the risks inherent in the experimental procedure, as mandated by federal and state regulations. "We take a very serious view of this sort of thing—particularly not informing the patient. He has the right to know if he wants to participate or if he doesn't. Most of them do, but the question is, How was he asked and did he actually read the thing? He [Chenin] signed it for surgery, so he knew about that.

"We're very concerned about patient protection. Please emphasize that the VA is miles above as far as informed consent is concerned. I assure you, the VA has led the way in informed consent."

And Dr. B.?

"He's the model," says Dr. Porter. "He dots every *i* and crosses every *t* since that's happened. He's very careful."

Dr. G., B.'s co-principal investigator in the project, apparently didn't fare as well. He was "forced" to resign, according to Porter, who adds, "It was really his research anyway."

The September 6 minutes of the Research and Education Committee make no mention of Dr. G. But they do reveal the fate of the study, and of its key proponent that day. "The recommendations of the Human Studies Sub-committee to withdraw approval from this project was not carried because of a tie vote," the official text, recorded and signed by Dr. Robert W. Porter, shows. Instead, the study "is suspended until such time as Dr. B. specifically requests the committee to consider it further."

A few months later, with committee sanction, Dr. B.—without Dr. G. and without Kenneth Chenin—was back in the hypertension and propranolol business.

In all, Dr. B. was associated with no less than thirteen research projects for the twelve months ending June 30, 1973. In nine of them, he is listed as principal investigator. Most of the studies concerned cardiovascular problems, including one that examined the effects of freeway travel on angina pectoris.

A half-dozen years later, Dr. Porter, sitting stiffly in the second-floor conference room of the chief of staff in the same building where Kenneth Chenin died, gathers up the material he retrieved from the file in order to refresh his memory about the case.

"I feel very comfortable in this hospital," he says.

Dr. Porter may feel at ease there, but more than fifty sworn affidavits suggest that that is not a universal emotion at the Long Beach VA and other VA medical facilities. The notarized statements contain three major themes: feeling pressured to participate in experiments, lack of information pertaining to the risks involved, and lack of clarity about the patient's right to withdraw at any time from the research.

The affidavits were acquired by the Institute for the Study of Medical Ethics, a Los Angeles–based, national volunteer non-profit group of health workers that began to investigate the question of informed consent after learning about the Chenin situation from a VA physician who requested anonymity. The institute, which numbers among its members doctors, nurses, lawyers, and lay people, is not opposed to the role of human experimentation in the progress of modern science. It does, however, "aim to ensure that the subjects . . . are not abused and that their rights are established and protected."

In pursuit of those goals, the institute was a key factor in the passage in 1978 of California's AB 1752, a law which for the first time in the state required that informed consent be obtained from a person before participation in a medical experiment.

In order to determine the extent of the allegations, the group placed a classified ad in the Los Angeles *Times.* "We quickly discovered that the VA was a source of a large number of these abuses," says Tom Armistead, thirty-two, the institute's former research director and one of its founders.

Armistead swiftly followed up and documented the stories.

"I think a lot of people in the VA, and other experimental situations, don't realize fully what they are getting themselves into. Even when patients are given a consent form to sign, that's not a fully informed consent because they'll just sign anything, especially if they're given a little pressure—'Hey, listen, we don't have time. Just sign these things . . .' "

Armistead, the son of an air force colonel, is not alone in his perspective. In fact, some high VA officials agree with him. One of them is the Manhattan VA's Tom Sherwood, who contends there are several intertwined layers wrapped around the issue.

"There must be a healthy respect and dignity for the patient," he says. "But there's only one way you can have that—if you're clear about who you are. . . . If you know that you are a physician, a nurse, a hospital aide, and your job is such that the patient comes first, then you don't have any problems. That's the problem with our government. They think they come first. They think their research comes first. They think what they do comes before the patient.

"So, therefore, when the doctor comes on the ward, the patient doesn't see it that way. 'I'm boss,' the doctor tells him. 'Do this like I say, or else.' Or, 'I'm going to do a certain procedure.' No informed consent. He doesn't tell the patient what it is. What is the definition of informed consent? Informed consent means you must tell him the risk. You must tell him why you're doing it. You must tell him what you expect to achieve by doing it. You must tell him the long- and short-range risks. You must tell him who's doing it, and who the team is.

"You must be prepared to speak to him about your qualifications if he asks. This is informed consent. You must give him the option to speak to it. If he doesn't understand it, you have the responsibility to get him to understand it. If he doesn't speak English, then you've got a responsibility to see that someone who speaks his language tells him what's going on. That's what I'm talking about."

Dr. Paul East, the English physician and attorney who heads up the VA's Medical-Dental education division, puts it much more succinctly.

"Consent forms are an abomination," he says in his D.C.-modulated British accent. "Patients are not consenting when they sign a consent form. There is no such thing as informed consent."

Recent statistics come close to bearing him out.

Almost 28 percent of the patients interviewed by the National Academy of Sciences for its 1977 report, *Biomedical Research in the Veterans Administration,* were not aware they had agreed to participate in a medical research study *even though signed consent forms were a part of each patient's record.* At least 20 percent of the patients interviewed had "very little or no idea of what the research was about," while about 12 percent "gave a reasonably complete and lucid account of the purpose or nature of the research." On the other hand, 95 percent of those responding said they "felt free to refuse research participation" and perceived it as being "purely voluntary."

At the time of the study, 1973, NAS reports that 2,547 out of 3,658 VA investigators said they used human subjects in their research. In addition, it was estimated that 17,500 VA patients were taken into research projects between February 1 and March 31, 1975—only a two-month period.

All the more reason why NAS worried that recently implemented, more restrictive VA guidelines "hadn't been disseminated or put into operation at some hospitals. This got the committee concerned about the adequacy of procedures pertaining to the obtaining of consent from patients for participating in research."

The concerns, apparently, were well founded.

On March 30, 1978, Clarice Anderson, fifty-two, of Santa Monica, California, swore in an affidavit for the Institute for the Study of Medical Ethics,

In February or March of 1977, while staying at Brentwood VA Hospital recovering from a nervous breakdown, a certain doctor asked me to take an experimental drug that he was doing research on. I was in terrible condition, upset, nervous, and overdrugged. I had been given so many drugs that I was confused about what was going on and I didn't want to take any more, especially one that had not been proven for human use.

I refused to take it. The doctor kept pestering me to take it, and I kept refusing him. Twice he called me into his office and demanded that I sign a consent form so that he could give me the drug. I kept refusing.

He kept this pressure up daily until finally I gave in, and signed the consent form, which said something like I knew that I was volunteering for an experiment. I do not remember any mention of potential side effects. The doctor told me that no one had ever been harmed by this drug [unknown name].

I took this pill for a few days. I don't know if this drug caused it, but I felt like I was dying, crying a lot, overmedicated, and very upset during this time. I felt pressured into this experiment. I was pushed until finally I felt I had to sign. There was no informed consent.

On April 26, 1979, Verlin Belcher, a Vietnam veteran from Gary, Indiana, swore in an affidavit for his Chicago lawyers

That on Thursday, April 19, 1979, the affiant [Belcher], together with one Jerry Wilson, a veteran . . . , and one James Hencin, another veteran, . . . were admitted to the Hines Veterans Administration Hospital, Hines,

Illinois, for the purpose, as explained to each of us, by doctors at said hospital and others, of having a simple procedure known as a fat biopsy performed upon each of us [to test for Agent Orange exposure]; doctors at the hospital informed us that the procedure would involve making a small incision of approximately one inch in length, that the sutures required to close the incision would be minimal, and as few as a single stitch, and that we would be able to go home afterwards and return to our normal activities and duties immediately upon discharge from the hospital. . . .

That affiant believes he was given a local anesthetic, after being draped in the operating room; thereupon doctors performing the procedure made an incision into the lower left quadrant of his abdomen which was approximately five to six inches long, and of unknown depth which required numerous internal sutures and 13 external sutures to close.

That affiant was discharged and left the hospital during the evening of Friday, April 20, 1979, and has been in severe pain since, and has been unable to return to his working occupation of crane operator for Bethlehem Steel Corporation since said date.

That if the doctors would have informed affiant of the true nature of the procedure actually performed upon him, he would not have consented to it; in fact did not consent to the procedure actually performed upon him, and has been substantially damaged in his earnings, has been permanently disfigured, and has endured pain and suffering by reason thereof.

That affiant is informed and believes that James Hencin . . . was likewise misinformed or uninformed . . . [and] likewise since been unable to pursue his occupation of carpenter . . .

One day in May, Harry Elmer Kuszmaul, forty-four, of Bellflower, California, swore in an affidavit for the Institute for the Study of Medical Ethics,

I entered the Long Beach VA because of acute angina pectoris [severe chest pains] due to a Workman's Compensation accident which occurred at Rodac Pneumatic Corp. in the city of Carson.

After a few months of testing and research and trying various different types of medications, and after conferring with [the doctor] it was decided that I should have an experimental open-heart surgery. I was told that the odds were 95% in my favor. Because he was in charge of the cardiac research at the Long Beach VA and presented himself as infallible and totally competent, I consented to have this open-heart surgery.

I signed a standard surgical consent form [not one for the experiment] but I was so heavily sedated I could barely comprehend it. To my knowledge there was no mention of potential risks or side effects. . . . Approximately 30 days after the surgery, I had a mild cardiac infarction [heart attack], the first one I had ever had. Subsequently, I have had two others. . . . If I had been properly informed of the potential side effects of the experiment I would never have consented to surgery.

"When people die or their condition worsens as the result of experimentation," says Tom Armistead, "it's too gross not to be looked at. If the guidelines were truly enforced—the bill we passed or the HEW guidelines—a lot less problems would occur.

"Why does it happen? I would have to surmise one thing: These people are getting their medical care for free. Medical experimentation needs to be done for various reasons and you put them both together and you get the current situation.

"If people were paying a lot of money, you could bet your bottom dollar they'd take more care of them. They probably wouldn't use them as guinea pigs. Very few people who are paying for their medical care get selected out as guinea pigs. So we use poor people at teaching hospitals. We use people at VA hospitals. I think the main thing is that they have to do these experiments, they want to do these experiments, and the people are right there—sign 'em up."

"The concept of informed consent is a troublesome one," reports Columbia University sociologist Dr. Bernard Barber. "The investigator wants enough subjects and is afraid of scaring them."

"The researchers want to minimize the number of people who will object to the research," says Armistead. "One way to do that is by using poor people or veterans who can't go somewhere else for their medical care. Hell, if you're sick and someone promises you help with a new pill or operation, it's very hard to say no."

Especially if you have nowhere else to go. The alliance among the VA, teaching institutions, and medical researchers works to the disadvantage of patients whose dependent financial status and lack of medical insurance ensure a stable cadre of "cases" to work on, Armistead says. They are physically and, often, emotionally depleted by age and the accumulated debilitation of war experiences where time has finally taken its terrible toll.

"The veterans experimented on are just the opposite of the highly qualified, well-known doctors," Armistead points out. "Poor people. Uneducated. They come to the VA because they can't afford to go anywhere else. They're the perfect class of people.

"The analogy is, of course, in pre-Nazi and Nazi Germany, where they started singling out various social classes, and they would start singling out the thieves, the retarded, the socially unfit, the sick. And these would be the people that everyone could agree upon as being, well, unproductive to society, of no value. These were the people targeted for experimentation and, ultimately, extermination. I've heard people say these poor veterans —especially the drunks, the hard to deal with—are a drain on our resources. If that's so, then what comes next?"

Indeed, "informed consent" as an ethical scientific-medical code of conduct emerged from the post–World War II Nuremberg trials, where medical experimenters were sentenced to death for their crimes against humanity. There were no such things as informed consent forms then.

Armistead suggests there is a lesson to be learned from all that. He thinks the VA central office should make it clear that it intends to enforce its patient protection regulations. "I think if they came down and said, 'Hey, listen, we're serious about this. We're getting too much flak from the public and some of you guys are costing us money in lawsuits'—then they'd get straight about this. A few large lawsuits would be very therapeutic."

Armistead is certain the abuses are widespread. "There's too many other things happening in other areas of the country for me to think that it's isolated here in one part of the country."

Terry Moakley is proof of that, even without the experimentation.

Moakley, a former marine lance corporal, is a wheelchair-bound quadriplegic who damaged his sixth cervical vertebrae in a diving accident. On one of the pale blue walls in his Eastern Paralyzed Veterans of America office in New York, where he is Barrier-Free Design Director for the group, is a Certificate of Appreciation from the New York State Advocate for the Disabled.

Moakley is a good-looking man, well dressed with red tie, matching shirt, and gray slacks. In 1975, he had kidney stones removed at the Bronx (Kingsbridge) VA Medical Center.

"Another couple of months later, in January, '76, it was the day after New Year's," he recalls, "for some reason I just stopped being able to pass water completely. I was told that will happen sometimes after a major kidney surgery like I just had. So I checked in about the second of January and they did about a week's worth of tests, different kind of tests to determine exactly what the problem was.

"And I was presented with an alternative—an operation, which is known as a transurethral resection. They simply cut a muscle in the bladder in order to enable you to void. It was either that or be on an in-dwelling catheter for the rest of my life.

"I didn't want that, so I asked the doctor—I can remember, on three different occasions—if this operation was going to have any effect on my sexual function. And on each occasion—and a couple of times my wife was there—he said, 'No. It shouldn't be any problem at all.' On all three occasions, he was very, very definite about it. He said there would be no change at all in the sexual function.

"So I had the operation and that was the end of my sexual function. He was wrong."

Moakley, who has a master's degree in English literature, stops for a moment to take a brief phone call. He lights a Newport, and continues.

"I went back two months subsequent to the operation to talk to the doctor about it. He was a resident, which is one of the real problems I find with the whole set-up there. It's a teaching hospital. You never get the same doctors, except on the spinal-cord ward. Also, they are relatively young doctors, new doctors.

"He told me he didn't understand why that function didn't

come back and he did research and he didn't find anything in the research as to why it should happen. I never really got any good answers from him . . . only that he didn't know why. He told me to try some different things, different procedures, which I tried and tried and which had no effect whatsoever. I've been living with this for three or four years and I've had a series of urinary tract infections—a couple, not many. And I just decided last spring that with everything that happened to me on the urological ward up there, I am not going to that hospital anymore."

In May, Moakley visited the Castle Point VA in Newburgh because he had heard good things about a female urologist there.

"I thought if I had gone back to the Bronx it would have been a new doctor and I would have to go through the whole history again and I just didn't want that. The urologist explained to me the physiological reason, probably why I lost my sexual function, which was never explained to me at the Bronx at all."

She also told him his problems probably stemmed from an incision made during the operation.

"I don't think that it was an error. The urologist at Castle Point told me that in eighty percent of these operations, there's no change at all. In ten percent, for some reason, a patient's sexual function will even get better as a result of this operation, and in another ten percent it will just diminish or completely end.

"She said that it is physiological, not psychological. There's no doubt about that. She didn't go so far as to say that he cut too much or he cut too deep or anything, but she said that the reason was probably the fact that the blood vessels were cut."

Although the bungled results of the operation remain, Moakley does not intend to pursue it any further.

"The doctor at Castle Point has been a urologist for a number of years," he says. "I don't know how many. But the doctor who did the operation on me in the Bronx was a resident, which means that he was practicing for only two or three years. There's no doubt in my mind that it was lack of informed consent. There's just no doubt about that."

Despite the fact that Bronx, Long Beach, and other VA officials strenuously deny the allegations of poor or nonexistent informed consent procedures and resultant abuses, the VA central office, tucked away in Washington, D.C., knows better. And it apparently makes no distinction between the veteran deciding whether to become involved in some research study and the veteran choosing among a variety of treatment modalities for the improvement of his health, as in Moakley's case.

In a statement as amazing for its between-the-lines candor as much as for its outright admission of complicity and culpability in the abusive, perhaps criminal, handling of unnumbered thousands of experimented-upon veteran-patients, the VA laid it on the line to its more than two hundred directors of medical centers, regional offices, domiciliaries, and outpatient clinics around the country. Writing in the March 22, 1979, Circular 10-79-58, a kind of irregular memo to selected VA staff in the field and not for general public distribution, Dr. Donald L. Custis, deputy chief medical director (since promoted to chief medical director) summarizes the most "Frequently Identified Inspector General Audit Deficiencies."

The audit, Custis gently explains, "is an assessment of how well VA medical centers comply with established agency guidelines in accomplishing assigned missions." Deficiency No. 8, therefore, gives the lie to the smugness with which the VA reflexively dismisses anguished complaints of "guinea pig" research or, even, uninformed clinical surgery.

Labeled "Consent Forms," it reads,

Controls should be strengthened to ensure proper completion and maintenance of consent forms. In *many* instances these forms are either not being completed or only partially completed. For example—the operation and/or procedure to be performed is not written in layman's terms [as required]. Without an appropriately completed form, the Medical Center cannot be assured that the patient *fully understands and voluntarily gives informed consent.* [Italics added.]

"I don't think people would get away with treating paying patients the way they treat veterans," insists Armistead. "And yet, the veterans *have* paid. They've paid in service to their country and they were promised this medical care, if not directly, at least through implications they would get it. "I think free medical care should be a drawing point and it should be medical care we as a nation are proud of. And that means respecting the rights of people, not violating them by pressuring them into operations they don't need or experiments they don't want, and which aren't even explained to them. The VA should do better than that."

As Dr. Custis's memo suggests and even casual observation supports, the issue of informed consent and its attendant ramifications has in fact become a major concern for the VA, involving large chunks of time from the agency's Office of the Inspector General (IG). Headed by Allan L. Reynolds, a certified public accountant with twenty-five years of government service, the IG was established on January 1, 1978, several months prior to congressional legislation that mandated the creation of inspector general positions in federal agencies.

The VA points out that its concerns were so overriding that it established the IG post before it was required. That's true, but a close look suggests that perhaps the agency, increasingly under fire for alleged abuses ranging from being a major supplier of illicit drugs in parts of the system to accusations that it was hiring too many foreign-language doctors, was more derelict than others in ferreting out and correcting problems.

In its November 1976 report, for example, the General Accounting Office, the government's fiscal watchdog agency, noted that the VA had the fewest auditors per dollar expended and per staff employed of any of the forty-nine federal audit agencies studied. In addition, the GAO said, the audit activities were not linked with the investigative activities in any kind of joint effort to combat waste, mismanagement, and fraud. One result was that VA facilities had no systematic review of their operations.

"If you were a hospital director, you could expect to be audited once every ten to fifteen years at most," says Reynolds, swept out in the Reagan takeover that promised new IGs "meaner than a junkyard dog." The Albuquerque VA, for instance, had not had a full management audit for twenty-five years, despite having a history of fraud and mismanagement. The audit done in 1980 found missing, incomplete, and blank consent forms throughout the surgical records.

Another result was that the broad area of quality of medical care had never been regularly examined by the VA in any comprehensive way, even though it frequently trumpeted the news that a major priority of its operation was to oversee conditions in the medical centers to make certain that veterans received the best possible care and treatment. Now, however, the IG is in place with its 340 auditors (it had 102 in 1977), and systematic reviews of each hospital are planned for three-year cycles (every five years for regional offices). With its major focus on prevention, according to Reynolds, the IG is equipped to handle instances of fraud, waste, and mismanagement.

There is no question that an independent Inspector General, reporting directly to the VA administrator but separate from him, was needed. For the first six months of its existence, October 1, 1978–March 31, 1979, the IG's office obtained twenty-eight convictions in the areas of fraud and theft, resulting in the recovery of $173,364.

Noting that the completed audits have resulted in "some significant findings and recommendations," the IG's first semiannual report further enthuses that "it is noteworthy that none [of the findings] reveals a significant short fall in the quality of service provided the veterans, a significant short fall in achieving desired program results, non-compliance with statutory requirements, or serious danger to health or safety."

The key phrase here is "significant short fall." There is, says Reynolds, none of them, while there are "some significant findings." The distinction is not explained. In any case, the following are some of what Inspector General Reynolds considers *not* to be significant short falls:

VA Medical Center Brooklyn, New York
We found a lack of retrospective medical care audits, over 600 delinquent hospital summaries and operations reports, and excessive lengths of stay in medical and surgical services.

Surveys by the Joint Commission on Accreditation of Hospitals, Systematic External Review Program staff and other surveyors in the two years preceding the audit contained 146 recommendations for improvements at the medical center. We found approximately 60 percent of these not implemented.

Outstanding bills for collection, for a total amount exceeding $70,000, showed no evidence of collection follow-up. In addition, vouchers for transfers between appropriations and/or funds, representing over $442,-000 due the VA, showed no attempts to collect. The documents involved included several outstanding since 1971.

VA Medical Center Saginaw, Michigan
The six-bed general purpose intensive care unit and the eight-bed respiratory intensive care unit were underused. During a 202-day period more than eight intensive care beds were needed only 31 days. The respiratory intensive care unit was not equipped to treat critically ill patients. By modifying plans for renovating the general purpose intensive care unit to include four beds for respiratory care patients, the respiratory intensive care unit could be closed at a savings of $100,000 per annum.

Space use was inadequate. There were five services with space deficiencies which adversely affected operations, yet there was unoccupied or underused space throughout the center. Two construction projects, one for $50,000 and one for $250,000, were cosmetic and did not provide adequate operating space for the Supply and Laboratory Services in spite of acknowledged space deficiencies.

Manila Grant-in-Aid Program
Expenses incurred by the VA at the outpatient clinic are not reimbursed at actual rates. Underpayments from grant funds to the VA in fiscal year 1978 totalled about $100,000.

University of Florida-Gainesville VA
The medical center was purchasing anesthesiology services via bimonthly purchase orders at a rate equivalent to $212,000 annually. The review determined that $84,084 of the proposed $212,000 cost was allowable. The remaining $127,916 represented proposed salary and fringe benefits exceeding University base rates for the same services. In essence the medical center was contracting with the Academic Enrichment Fund and not the University, since VA payments were made to an individual in the Anesthesiology Department for inclusion in the AEF.

The results of a desk review of a proposed fiscal year 1979 contract were issued on January 4, 1979, questioning approximately $150,000 of a proposed annual cost of $256,500. An unacceptable record of price negotiation was received on April 10, 1979, which did not show the disposition of the $150,000 questioned costs.

It is striking that nowhere in the findings and recommendations is there an attempt to place specific responsibility for a facility's problems on any individual. Nowhere is the recommendation made to fire, fine, suspend, or even slap the wrist of *someone, somewhere* for allowing these nonsignificant shortfalls to occur. One of the recommendations to correct the lack of implementation of improvements at the Brooklyn VA, for example, is the directive to "establish controls to monitor progress toward implementation of recommendations." The recommendation at another office for maintaining a register of fee-basis physicians (after abuses were uncovered) is, believe it or not, "Maintain a register of fee-basis physicians."

Reynolds says he is prohibited by the Privacy Act from designating specific accountability in the report. Additionally, the "type of almost absolute personal accountability/responsibility which would give rise to such recommendations is rare. Often responsibility is shared, sometimes in a widely diffused manner, or involving other federal, state, or local organizations. In such cases, lines of accountability become very blurred." Nonetheless, Reynolds reports that at the Brooklyn VA, for one, "none of these findings resulted in recommendations for disciplinary action, nor did responses to these recommendations from the responsible VA departments and staff offices indicate that disciplinary action had been taken."

Across the country, in California, disciplinary action was likewise avoided in an area of which Reynolds and his auditors were undoubtedly unaware. Medical training has not come under the same kind of scrutiny the inspector general's office has afforded other components of the VA, but the potential effect on patient care is certainly not any less. Medical residents at VA hospitals are paid to learn about the various aspects of patients' illnesses under the supervision of a qualified physician. It is a clinical experience, though veterans like Moakley might argue otherwise.

Yet at at least one VA hospital, and, if history is any guide, others as well, residents are going beyond their authorized mandate.

"Some residents are doing research at the San Francisco VA, against contractual and VA regulations," asserts Dr. William Hamilton, chairman of the University of California–San Francisco's Department of Anesthesiology and chief of staff at the affiliated VA there.

It's more than one department, he adds, declining to identify them other than to say his isn't on the list. Asked how they get away with it, Dr. Hamilton, at the medical school for thirteen years, laughs. "You probably went over the speed limit on your way here today."

Actually, I had walked to his office.

[C]ertain criteria must be met. The patient must be well-hydrated and well-nourished, and there must be reasonable standards of personal cleanliness, particularly if the patient is unable to care for himself. . . . There is no reason for a patient to be constantly worried about his or her physical condition.
—*From* The Aging Veteran: Present
and Future Medical Needs *(VA
report)*

5

GROWING OLD WITH, AND AT, THE VA

Currently, almost one-half of all American males over the age of twenty are veterans, with an average age of forty-seven. By 1990, barring a war, 18 million veterans will comprise more than half of all U.S. men sixty-five years and older—while the total number of veterans will have declined. That represents a tripling of the number of post-sixty-five former servicemen since the mid-1970s, all within a fifteen-year span.

By 1995, the figures will rise in excess of 60 percent of the total. Veterans will therefore constitute the major proportion of the male aged population during the remainder of the twentieth century. By the year 2000, the VA projects a need for 120,000 beds. That's 33 percent more than it has now.

It is a population growing progressively larger, older, and sicker.

You would think, then, that the VA would have been feverishly dedicating a large segment of its resources and committing a good deal of its energies to ensuring that a solid, humane program is being built now to be firmly in place when the brunt of the need is predicted to arise.

Cliff and Ruth Carroll thought so, too.

Cliff, a retired supervisor after thirty-seven years at Kraft Cheese, is the kind of guy who says, "You know, it's the veterans who should be getting help, getting care.

"They deserve it. If it weren't for them, where would we be? I don't know if it's patriotism, or what—but when I hear the 'Star-Spangled Banner' or see a big flag or hear a parade, I get all tingly inside. The veteran, whatever his age, if he needs help, he should get it. But they don't seem to be getting it."

Carroll, sixty-one, though briefly in the army some thirty-five years ago, is not talking about himself on a bright, obscenely hot, late Sunday morning in the San Fernando valley. He has just spent a couple of hours indoors showing a visitor around, and now he is standing in the narrow circular driveway that fronts a squat one-story brick building at the Sepulveda VA Medical Center just north of Los Angeles. The two-year-old structure, dubbed "99" in a burst of bureaucratic imagination, is identified by the equally creative round orange and black sign pasted to its exterior. Off in the smog-fuzzed distance, what appear to be mountains gently vibrate in the hundred-degree man-made soup, outlining what was once the designated lair of one Charles Manson and his own covey of copyrighted polluted visions.

Inside the building, which contains the nursing home on this sprawling hospital campus, Mrs. Carroll's brother, Dale, is the responsibility of the U.S. Veterans Administration. Because they question the adequacy of that particular federal undertaking, the Carrolls maintain a very special rhythm to their lives, born of the timeless biblical mandate to care profoundly for thine own flesh and blood. And because, as orphans themselves, they know the vulnerability to which human beings without props are often subject, the Carrolls journey to Sepulveda weekly from their home in Buena Park, a round trip of seventy-five miles.

Cliff and Ruth Carroll have visited Dale every Saturday since

1973—except once, when Cliff attended a company picnic. Their brother's keepers, they would mount the freeways regularly even if the VA did its appointed job. As it is, they bring along foodstuffs, clean clothes, and other paraphernalia of well-being. Today, a Sunday two weeks before the beginning of autumn, is an exception. But the break in routine, at the request of an interested chronicler they have never met before, does not find a coincident respite inside the sturdy walls of No. 99.

"Once," says Ruth Carroll, "we came to visit and Dale's arm was red, like a bad sunburn. We discovered it dressing him to take him home one weekend. It turned out to be an infected elbow. The staff denied knowing anything about it. That was at two P.M. The nurses said they checked him at noon and saw nothing. We had to take him to the emergency room. It needed to be lanced."

He has also had an unnoticed broken collar bone. When the Carrolls express interest in his condition, says Mrs. Carroll, "They tell me, 'Why are you so concerned, he's only your brother.' "

Dale Williams, fifty-five years old and a World War II army infantryman and signal corpsman, can no longer defend himself. In fact, he is unable to communicate his simplest needs, much less explain in detail a nurse's negligence or a doctor's arrogance. Dale Williams is in the later stages of Huntington's chorea, a degenerative nervous system disease that renders its victims, like Dale, speechless and helpless. He is at the mindless mercy of a body once vigorous enough to carry arms for his country but now out of control, a body that cannot even coordinate itself to accurately place a cigarette in its mouth.

He is, moreover, a VA statistic, one of the hundreds of thousands who will be over sixty-five in 1990.

A VA report on the subject, *The Aging Veteran: Present and Future Medical Needs,* states:

The goal of nursing home care is to provide a framework of therapeutic services for restoring patients to optimal health in facilities which meet modern environmental standards and safety. . . . It is extremely important that staffing be adequate both as to numbers and mix of types of personnel. When the workload is heavy there is inadequate time to develop interpersonal relationships with and support for these isolated patients for whom this is a major component of therapy. . . . Through training, counseling and assessment the personnel will be kept aware of the components of a good environment, and will be encouraged to maintain the highest standards.

The manual was written in 1977, the same year Dale Williams was moved into the new Sepulveda nursing home. Despite its characterization by the VA as a "comprehensive report" that "may serve as a basic resource document for planning for the care of aging veterans for the next two decades," it apparently hasn't yet been circulated in Building 99.

Nursing-home care for veterans is authorized under PL 88-450, passed in August 1964. The nursing home is for veterans who are not acutely ill and not in need of hospital care. They do, however, require a great deal of skilled nursing attention and lesser amounts of medical and associated services for protracted periods of time, according to the VA.

Generally, therefore, VA nursing homes are adjacent to full-service VA hospitals. Length of stay is related to the individual's needs and is not time-limited. In 1978, ninety-one nursing home units were in operation, 11,671 patients were treated, and the average number of operating beds was 7,884.

"With the veteran population growing older all the time," says former New York Congress member Lester Wolff, "there is an urgent need for expanded nursing home care." He adds, "Unless the VA corrects some of these problems, it will be fair game for those who want to destroy it."

Ruth Carroll wonders whether that hasn't already begun to happen.

She has just greeted Dale in his room, patting his stubble-bearded face and talking quietly to him. The room, toward the back of the building, has brown and white walls. It is pleasantly furnished with two beds with made-up green bedspreads, a semi-private bathroom, and a door leading to an outside patio. The halls are sparkling clean, the floors waxed to a high shine that accents the bright, bold, orange and blue colors that seem to be everywhere.

It feels new and very well cared for.

The floor in Dale's room is dull in comparison, obviously not recently waxed, with dirt and debris scattered here and there. It's been that way for weeks, says Ruth Carroll. As she says hello to her brother, she and her husband quickly and with familiarity set about to do the chores. By now, after all those Saturdays, they have the routine efficiently organized.

While Cliff hangs up the freshly cleaned and ironed clothes they brought with them, and removes the week's accumulation of dirty garments, Ruth feels around Dale's pajama-clad body to make sure he is physically okay. She no longer takes any chances.

Then Dale's sister plugs in an electric razor and shaves off his seven-day growth of beard, washes his hair and face with a nice-smelling lotion, clips his toenails, lightly sands the underside of his feet, checks his closet, holds a small can of tomato juice for him to drink, and, when he is all done, gently brushes his hair into place.

It is accomplished with warmth and care and feeling. "They never do any of this," she turns and says. "It only took me ten minutes. That's too much for them."

He is presentable now, and Ruth rolls Dale in his wheelchair out to the hallway toward the home's common room. On the way, Cliff says that once they found caked shit under Dale's fingernails, which the staff had neglected to clean up. "And," he adds, looking sadly at the depleted figure being slowly pushed along the cleansed Congoleum path, "his wheelchair gets dirty all the time. We've had to hose it down. Like one old man said to us, 'They never clean your wheelchair—unless you die.'"

Dale's image is picked up by the portable black-and-white TV monitor left unattended at the nurses' station. The image fades to another: a tall, skinny, rickety man shuffling down the empty hallway with an unsteady cane. No one, on this deserted Sunday, is at the television set to note his progress, or the strength or weakness of his gait.

In the large common room, a becalmed sea of some thirty or forty wrinkled vets in wheelchairs is watching the Steelers and Oilers on a donated color TV. They are silent and motionless, obediently sitting in front of the glowing tube, its fickle portraits of virility flashing by with the coveted football or brutally nailing a high-stepping running back.

It is not clear how many are actually paying attention to the contest. Some are staring off into space, some are sleeping, some drooling.

There is no movement as the second quarter ends.

The score at half time is Steelers 9, Oilers 0.

There are only a half-dozen family visitors in evidence today. Flanked by colorful murals looking onto a dirty floor that was just mopped, the room, with a large American flag on a stand project-ing above everything and everybody, is being painted for the pa-tients' enjoyment. Mr. Carroll lights a cigarette for Dale and places it in his mouth. Mrs. Carroll opens some food, and begins to feed her brother. Pretty girls in flimsy outfits cavort across the half-time spectacle on the television.

"One time," Cliff Carroll says, "Dale told them his leg hurt, after falling down at breakfast. But they didn't do anything until hours later. His leg got swollen. One of the janitors told us he fell on the wet floor after it was mopped. He said he saw it happen. A nurse spoke to the janitor, and after that, he said he couldn't talk about it, he didn't see anything. The leg was broken in two places. They put Dale in a cast and in a wheelchair for one year, with no therapy or nothing.

"We always wonder when we come here—what are we going to find out today?"

The Carrolls bear the burden of others, too.

About a year ago, a patient was mistakenly locked in the rest-room all night. "They found him there when they opened up in the morning," Cliff says.

The heat is beating down on the rented green Pinto in the nursing home driveway. Sun rays are radiating off the sign that identifies Building 99. Cliff Carroll, a mild-mannered man, dressed for the southern California weather, is still bewildered by it all. He looks toward the place where his brother-in-law lives and says, quietly, "They think about the veterans once a year—on Memorial Day—then they forget about them."

He pauses. He seems to pay no attention to the ovenlike air.

"I say we should do what we can for Dale while he's still here alive. What good is it if you don't and he's gone and then you say we should have done this or that? Do what you can now, and then you have no regrets."

Inside, in the coolness, Ruth Carroll is tending to her brother, and thinking about how he no longer looks forward to returning to the nursing home after a weekend with the Carrolls in Buena Park. "When Dale is with us at home, after I get him to bed," Ruth Carroll says, her eyes clouding over, "I just sit there and cry to think somebody has to go through all of that like he does."

She turns her head away.

"What a terrible shame," she says

The shame, unfortunately, is extensive.

The VA admits there is an "acute shortage of nursing home facilities for the placement of veteran patients." Further, in the homes that do have openings, "the quality of many of these beds is so poor that there may be difficulty in finding adequate placements as the community load also rises." In other words, the good beds that do exist will be fought over by veterans and nonveterans from the community.

But nursing homes are not the only places for the VA's elderly.

There is a second extended-care component charged with the treatment of older veterans. It is the domiciliary program. Currently, there are fifteen domiciliaries, or doms, which in 1978 treated 17,275 veterans. (There is also one independent domiciliary in White City, Oregon.) The newest dom, a 200-bed replacement facility at Wood, Wisconsin, opened January 1980. It is the first new dom in twenty-seven years. The oldest, at Bath, New York, was built in the 1890s. It is still in use.

Domiciliary patient-members, as they are called, generally are drawn from three groups: the socially disaffiliated, mainly chronic alcoholics or former psychiatric patients who are relatively young; patients with primarily medical or surgical diagnoses who usually are older and require a sheltered environment for physical reasons; and a small group with good potential for rehabilitation, but who need some protective ambulatory care.

Domiciliaries are actually the original programs in the VA and were part of legislation in 1866 that established Soldiers Homes for disabled veterans. Perhaps as a result, many Americans persist in seeing the entire VA system, not just the doms, as a place that takes care of old soldiers.

The doms, admittedly, are not the VA's pride and joy.

"Most [domiciliaries] have serious life-safety and privacy deficits," the VA's *Aging Veteran* reports. "Of the 10,000 remaining domiciliary beds, it has been found by survey that only ten percent could be brought to acceptable standards by renovation at less than the costs of new construction."

That's bad enough. What's worse is that the patient-member, once he's in, can't get out—unless he slugs the director or sets fire to his room. According to the VA's *Aging Veteran,* "At present, there is no mechanism by which patients can be discharged from the domiciliary except for violation of domiciliary regulations."

Just to make certain the world knows that the VA, after all, does have some vague notion of what modern-day health care is about, the report adds, "If the rehabilitative potential of the domiciliaries is to be realized, there must be provision for a maximum domiciliary benefit concept, comparable to that of maximum hospital benefits, leading to discharge."

In 1975, fully one-third of those leaving the VA's domiciliaries were classified as "irregular discharges"—patients in violation of dom procedures or otherwise removing themselves without official sanction (the other two-thirds knocked around various parts of the VA system). Though the 1977 National Academy of Sciences' comprehensive study of VA facilities found domiciliary programs to be "residential, rather than rehabilitative" and the medical service "adequate," it was critical of the overall atmosphere. "The individual programs directed toward rehabilitation are too few and too thinly staffed to be effective in reaching their avowed goals."

"The social climate of the domiciliaries reflects an institutional pattern of formal behavior, best described as benevolent paternalism, and rated as inadequate by the site visitors. The domiciliaries provide austere homes for a disaffiliated, infirm population of men," the report concludes.

"The VA," says Lester Wolff, "has not really gotten hold of the difference between domiciliary care and the normal hospital care of a patient."

No one knows that better than the occupants of the doms themselves.

"The domiciliary gave me no psychological therapy, gave me no psychiatric therapy, and it gave me no aphasic training. They give no therapy at all. I have three broken teeth. That's for eight months now. I haven't had them fixed. When you ask for something, they resent you asking for what is yours. We're supposed to have new beds and new mattresses and new lockers. I've been denied that.

"They restrict us getting good food. Now, to give an example, the dom is supposed to get two hundred and twenty pounds of tomatoes for a week. And we get not even one-quarter of one tomato a week with our meals. We get very little fresh fruits and fresh vegetables. Most of it is old food that we have.

"It's not like we used to get, years before. The salads have secondary lettuce. We have to sort out the old parts and throw it away. We don't know what happens to the good stuff that we're supposed to get. Most of the meat is old. You can see it. It's crumbled up, so you know it's not really a fresh cut of meat.

"The men are supposed to get fed according to their diets. But the dietitians are never there to oversee it. They just give me what they want. If it's something I can't eat, I just don't eat it. It just doesn't seem possible, but it does happen that way."

Irwin Tyson, fifty-five, is sitting in the basement of a building on the grounds of the Los Angeles (Wadsworth) VA Medical Center domiciliary. Tyson, in and out of the dom over the past several years, has a scar over the left side of his head, the result of fourteen hours of brain surgery in 1959. The surgeon removed 100 cc.'s of brain tissue, causing a loss in memory ability, or aphasia.

Dressed in a white sweat shirt with short sleeves, white socks, and blue jeans with a one-inch light blue stripe running down the side, he is describing his experiences at the deteriorating facility. It would be hard to imagine a more depressing place. More than half the aging buildings are shuttered for a variety of safety reasons. Its 68.7 percent occupancy rate in 1977 was the lowest of all the doms, most of which had levels of 90 percent and above. One year later, the occupancy rate had moved up to 89.3 percent by the simple device of shuttering more beds.

The grounds border on the ill-kept, and the occupied buildings are dingy and getting worse. Officials and veterans alike say it was one of the nicer doms at the turn of the century.

Tyson is one of those patient-members who has been discharged for disciplinary reasons. He says it's because the administration objects to his complaints about the abuses suffered by the men. When the dom kicks him out, he lives in his wheezing 1956 white Chevy stepvan. At one stretch, he called the rolling, windowless vehicle home for four years. The van is crammed full with Tyson's years of accumulated survival trappings. On the outside, a propane tank hugs the rear bumper and spare tires are affixed to a rooftop luggage rack.

Physically, he looks like the truck's owner. His salt-and-pepper beard is sort of overgrown but neat. Tiny hairs grow upward and out from his bushy eyebrows, rising above his brown-tinted glasses. Bald, he could easily be mistaken for an aging Hunter Thompson. "There's a tremendous flow of pills out here," he says. "A lot of patients keep the drugs and then sell them."

Like all the doms, this one has some younger psychiatric patients mixed in with the elderly population. It also has, like all doms, "limited psychosocial and medical programs ... available," according to the VA's own account. To a large extent, then, the patient-members create their own activities to pass the time.

Some of them push drugs.

Others watch the passing scene.

"When I was here approximately two months," recalls Norbert Blank, a sixty-two-year-old former navy department engineer-technician and technical writer for Lockheed, "I was in the bingo room, and I noticed a guy getting up to change his bingo card between games.

"Now, when he got up, he had shit in the chair. He had defecated in his trousers and he had also urinated in his pants, and that was on the seat, I could see it, in terms of the full imprint of his pants. Anyway, he got up, walked up, and changed his card.

Meantime, another fella—one of the unusual ones around here, nattily dressed and clean—sat down in the same seat.

"Now you know that mess went all over his trousers. But he didn't know it. He wanted to talk to somebody who was sitting down there. He had a few words with him, and got up and went away. This other guy comes over with the change of bingo card, with his drawers full, sits right back down in the same seat again.

"But listen to this. About a week and a half later, I see this same character get aboard the elevator and turn around—I'm in the back of the elevator—and I'm looking right at his drawers, right at his pants. And there's a crap still in his pants. A week and a half later. That guy must have put those trousers on every single morning, every single day.

"That's how they take care of the people here."

Blank, four years in the army during the Second World War, is at the domiciliary recovering from a heart attack. He is a relative newcomer, having arrived six months earlier. But he is as bitter as any old-timer there, like Tyson sitting nearby in the dom basement.

"After my heart attack, I was not allowed out of the room, but I could get up from the bed and was allowed to go to the toilet, which was part of the room. This was in the cardiac unit at the hospital. The doctor had come over to me that morning and she just put her stethoscope over here, and here—just two spots. Boop. Boop. Then some guy called her over from the other side of the room, and she never come back after that.

"Later on in the day, the nurse says to me, 'You're going to be leaving here today.' I says, 'I'm going to be leaving here today?'

"She says, 'Yes, you're going over to the dom.'

"I said, 'I'm not supposed to even leave the room here. Do you know what happens to somebody who has to go over to the domiciliary?' She says, 'Yeah, you get fed over there, just like you do here.'

"They forget a patient like me gets fed in bed. I can't go walking around. I'm not allowed to. At the domiciliary, you have to go up to the mess hall. You get aboard a bus. You have to take the elevator or walk down the stairs, and walk up to where the bus is.

And then the bus takes you through the chuckholes up there to the mess hall.

"This is about two weeks after my heart attack. So I says to her, I'm not ready to leave. You better send a doctor over here. Anyone you can get a hold of. All the doctors are interns or residents, that's all they are. When I first went in there I had a good intern. I'll tell you what a good intern is. He used to come over to my bed and check me and ask me how I felt. He checked me out thoroughly, two or three times a day. Nothing unusual for him. Then he left.

"Anyway, I said I wasn't going to leave the hospital today. So the nurse and doctor come over and said, 'Oh, yes, you are.' And I said, 'You're not getting me out of here. I want to see your boss.'

"Well, they sent over in about two or three hours two other birdlegs, just interns, and they started in on me. 'Don't you feel good?' I says I feel as well as I can right now. And then they give me this old harassment, you know? 'Well, you would like to get out of here today, wouldn't you?'

"I says no. And they're trying to put words in my mouth. And then finally it dawned on me that they were just giving me some runaround. I said I want to speak to my psychologist there. I said, 'I don't want to speak anymore to you birds at all.' My blood pressure went way the hell up during that day. Boy, oh, boy, I think it hit a hundred and seventy. Went way up.

"The psychologist got me another week in there. I told him, 'These interns made me feel worse. What the hell's the matter with them? They want me to have another heart attack?' They made me feel horrible, just horrible."

Blank says things have deteriorated dramatically.

"Now, the elevators work sometimes. Other times, they're broken down. It's nothing unusual to have people tinkering with the elevators on and off, on and off all the time. You go into the latrine and you turn the water on and the drains are all stopped up. There's about one death a week here.

"And, oh, yeah, for instance, over at the hospital, they have a special person comes around and disinfects the bed, you know. But here, if anything happens, why, they just throw some clean linen on the bed, and it's ready for the next guy. You're treated as if you're a fifth- or sixth-class citizen. There's no privacy in this place, just nothing, nothing. You're treated as if you're on some kind of a prison farm. But I belong here. I'm a patient."

Meanwhile, back at VA headquarters, the agency is busy congratulating itself on its self-assessment as a coming leader in the field of geriatric health care. A "more therapeutically aggressieve [*sic*] use of the domiciliaries will be necessary to realize their potential" is the way the nation's cutting edge of farsighted medical programming feelingly puts it.

Never mind that the aged veteran has had to cope in the past with crumbling buildings, failing equipment, insensitive staff, faltering medical care—not to mention nonaggressive (nonexistent?) therapy—the VA is now marching forward with vigor.

Along with building its first new domiciliary in years, the VA forthrightly pursued its own mandate when, in 1978, it selected nine physicians for the Geriatric Fellowship Program, a two-year block of special training in geriatrics with emphasis on the care of veterans over age sixty-five. The program has been expanded to include twenty-four fellows.

Underpinning this move is the Geriatric Research, Education and Clinical Centers (GRECC) program, thought up in 1973. By 1975, the VA established the first GRECCs.

Tellingly, the GRECC idea grew out of the understanding that "despite the need for geriatric support for the growing number of aged individuals in the community, and the special need of the VA, there was a professional disinclination to become involved in this area," according to one VA report on the subject.

Aging never has been a glamorous area of medicine, nor a particularly lucrative one—hence the "professional disinclination." With little or no money flowing directly from federal or other coffers to subsidize the teaching of geriatrics, U.S. medical schools have wallowed at other troughs, specifically the VA and its passive acceptance of direction by the affiliated medical community.

The care of chronic, long-term patients—that is, geriatric medicine—has never been in the forefront of American medicine. Indeed, the VA–medical school affiliations exemplify this attitude. If American medical schools have any complaints about their sweetheart contract with the VA, it is that the VA, responsible for an increasing caseload of aging veterans and their unique problems, has too many chronic, debilitated, uninteresting patients. It is a surfeit for which their eager young students, awash with borrowed enthusiasm for the emergent, acutely ill veteran, see no reason to develop their growing skills.

"The medical schools are out to take good care of themselves," says Harvey Sapolsky, a professor of health policy at MIT. "They do a job on the VA. Clearly, it's a gold mine for them." Sapolsky, in fact, along with three colleagues, has offered a generalized blueprint for making the VA "the nation's model for long-term, chronic care and alcohol rehabilitation, problems that have been neglected by American medicine and are of special importance to veterans."

Writing in the *Journal of Health Politics, Policy and Law,* Michael Lipsky, Lawrence McCray, Jeffrey Prottas, and Sapolsky add, "The bulk of the VA's medical resources . . . is devoted to the care of acutely ill veterans suffering from non-service connected disease problems.

"Paralleling the rest of American medicine, the VA has focused on the more exotic while neglecting the more mundane in health care. It has, for example, excess capacity to do open heart surgery, a rare and expensive procedure, but is short of certain types of nursing-home beds, and of space in its alcohol rehabilitation programs."

Though congressional budget restrictions have placed heart surgery dollars at certain VA medical centers at a relative premium since those GAO-generated facts were issued, the thrust has remained the same. Compounding it is the VA's original impetus for suggesting the affiliation agreement: to lift its (accurate) image of medical inferiority by associating itself with the prestigious medical schools. Not only did this aid in the recruitment of physicians, according to Sapolsky *et al.*, but it also "served to legitimize the quality of care offered in the VA hospitals."

Thus, rather than upgrade its reputation by expanding the types of service needed by its unique consumer population, the

VA chose instead to increase its standing by affiliating with the high-gloss medical schools. This decision, a slap in the face to all the veteran stood for, insured a continuation of its movement away from direct patient care and toward an alignment with forces mandated otherwise, from a momentum of serving patients to the seeking of recognition by medical colleagues.

The veteran suffered tremendously as a result, and some of the fruits of that estrangement can be seen in the paucity of programs and planning for the aged veteran in particular. "It's a mixed bag," says Congress member Ray Roberts, powerful former chairman of the House Veterans' Affairs Committee. "Overall the affiliations are a plus—we're helping train doctors and the patients are getting care. But it's not without its drawbacks."

The VA, of course, could rightfully use the enormous leverage it has to force the medical schools to create geriatric programs and services. The GRECC program is a belated step in that direction. But the VA could certainly push the schools even farther: If they wished to continue partaking of the cornucopia of virtually no-strings-attached goodies, then the schools should start becoming responsive to the types of patients the VA does serve, rather than bemoaning the dearth of "interesting" cases it doesn't serve.

As Sapolsky *et al.* point out, the VA annually provides hundreds of millions of dollars in direct and indirect subsidies to the schools. And, of course, much-needed teaching "material." The medical schools cannot easily give up this largesse. But if they do, the VA can always go back to its original mandate: treating sick American veterans instead of providing good teaching cases. For if it's doctors you need, it costs far less to hire competent full-time VA physicians to staff hospitals across the board than it does to maintain the affiliation. Far less.

But the medical schools are not asleep. As the VA increases the ante, as it says it will, and makes more monies available for geriatric research and clinical programs, the medical schools, ever alert to sniff out the big bucks, will suddenly realize the enormous benefits to be gained by their students on the chronic wards. Indeed, some of the new doctors, once so trained, might even specialize in gerontology in their private practices.

Sic transit professional responsibility.

Max Cleland proudly notes that his 1978 budget request included funds for construction of domiciliaries at Dayton and Martinsburg and design funds for Bath. "At this rate of funding," he says, ". . . it will take until fiscal year 1995 to completely upgrade the domiciliaries."

"The administration is not really concerned with excellence of care," asserts the Reverend Ronald A. Gunton, the part-time chaplain and full-time union leader at the Bath, New York, VA Medical Center. The Bath facility has 800 domiciliary beds and 200 hospital beds.

"If they were concerned, they would have drastically higher-quality care. As it is, we're just warehousing the veterans here. It's just warm storage. The VA," he says, "it's hard to define it. Is it socialism or socialized medicine or a manifestation of national ineptitude—or both?"

"The VA has to use its leverage more adequately," suggests Jon Steinberg, the astute, knowledgeable top aide to Senator Alan Cranston. Cranston was the chairman of the Senate Veterans Affairs Committee.

"For example, geriatrics. That's a big issue for this country. Medical schools don't rotate their students through nursing homes, they don't see the older veteran as a priority. They're also not interested in alcoholism. We've got to get the medical educators more interested in those areas."

A report by the University of California–San Francisco School of Medicine Health Policy Program puts it differently. But the message is equally clear.

"Rightly or wrongly, it is the level of VA support of a medical school's program that is often the fundamental determinant of the VA's degree of influence on that school. A California hospital director said: 'If the VA puts a lot of money into a school program it has influence. Otherwise, all the rejects are sent to the VA.' "

The report adds that "the VA's ability to provide and continue such support should be directed not simply at reproducing more of what presently exists, but at providing incentives toward resolutions of the problems." The increase in the number of aged veterans in VA hospitals "may encourage medical schools to turn to community hospitals and other health care institutions as possible new training resources, thus, over the long term, diminishing the role of the VA in medical education unless its eligible patient population and the way it provides medical care also change."

Given the operative demographics and the medical school's needs (and greed), it's hard to take the predicted extortion attempt seriously.

But the stakes are serious enough. "If the VA is not part of the solution," the report admonishes, "it will be a significant part of the problem."

In 1978, in partial response to that clarion call, the VA designated eight facilities as sites of its fledgling attempt to lead the way for the reluctant medical schools. The search for a geriatric solution was officially underway.

Unfortunately, however, the problem may not have been clearly defined, or advertised.

Though Ruth and Cliff Carroll and Dale Williams, Irwin Tyson, and Norbert Blank probably don't know it, one GRECC is at Sepulveda, and another is at Wadsworth. No signs were posted, apparently.

I am the sunlight on ripened grain,
    I am the autumn rain:
When you awake in the morning hush
    I am the swift uplifting rush.
            —*Anonymous American soldier,*
            found in his camouflage fatigue
            pocket, KIA Vietnam, 1970

... last winter, when I traveled around to find some
of the men who had gone as boys to Vietnam, the
war did not seem to have ended after all. In fact, it
seemed obvious that no war ends until all the people who have participated in it have died or lost
their memories.
            —*Tracy Kidder, magazine writer,*
            Harvard graduate, Vietnam
            intelligence officer

6

THE POISON ORANGE

"Please forgive me for imposing upon your most valuable
time, but I have a problem I think you should be aware of" begins
a February 26, 1979, letter to Congressman Donald Ritter from an
Allentown, Pennsylvania, constituent.

I understand other persons in the Lehigh Valley have the same problem, but they stand alone, as I do, in receiving proper attention in the
matter.

I was poisoned by Dioxin while in Vietnam. I served with the Marines
in 1965. I was with an artillery unit near Danang. We got our drinking
water from the Danang River. I am convinced I was poisoned through
the water.

Some locations I visited during my tour were defoliated by 2-4-5-T [2,
4, 5-T] containing Dioxin.

The water tasted so badly, I rely on my thoughts of drinking the bitter
slime-like substance and thinking the water must be poison. The mess-
hall gave us Kool-Aid to put in the water to kill the dreadful taste. I recall

154

directing a letter to the Kool-Aid Co. telling them how thankful I was for their products as the water was unbearable without the Kool-Aid flavor.

I also recall never seeing a bird in the areas of Vietnam I traveled. I assume the defoliant killed the birds.

I saw a dog stagger from the bush one day as if he were mad—I killed the dog with my entrenching tool to prevent his infecting one of our Marines.

A few days later, I saw one of our own men with the same symptoms. He was choking to death and his body was in violent convulsions. I saw our Marines go completely mad all around me. I thought it was battle fatigue.

I saw a Vietnamese Major's baby with sores over its body and assumed it had cold sores. I had a rash on my body along with other Marines—we thought we had heat rash.

I lost 40 lbs. and thought it was related to the climate. When I returned to the States I had swelling in my knee joints and sharp pain in my upper legs. I was told by doctors that I had arthritis and rheumatism. I wore a cast on my right leg for months and finally the swelling went down.

I ran a 26 mile marathon in 1976, which was about five years after the cast was removed. I had no further trouble with my knee joints.

The Military sprayed over 50,000 tons of defoliant, Agent Orange, in our area. They defoliated 4,000,000 acres of jungle. The chemical was sprayed from boats and from aircraft.

I was not told by medical personnel when departing Vietnam that Dioxin contamination of the body creates mutations or malformed children. My daughter Marcelle Jeanne was born within 19 months after my return from Vietnam. She was born with numerous deformities.

She has a cleft palate; heart murmur; blind, deformed right eye; no right ear or canal; deformed jaw bone; club right foot, etc. . . . Marci has had over 40 doctors attend her since birth. She needs constant observation as one of her problems may cause a major health hazard and require immediate attention.

I have appealed to almost every agency in hopes of gaining protection for Marci. I have fought for the past ten years and my efforts have ended to no avail. Local agencies tell me I make too much money to qualify for aid. I work four jobs and can't afford to quit one to qualify for assistance.

I would like to direct your attention to the Dioxin spill in Seveso, Italy, during July of 1976. Many women were allowed to have abortions because the Italian Government realized Dioxin caused deformed children. At the time abortion was against the law in Italy. The women deciding against the abortions had babies with exact defects as my Marci.

I have enclosed a copy of a letter from the Veterans Administration dated June 4, 1975. The VA informs me Marci is not a veteran and is not covered for benefits.

I wrote President Nixon about my problem, he never answered, but I received a personal visit from the VA at my home. My wife and I finally ended up seeing a marriage counselor as a result of the visit.

A letter dated 28 Aug '78 is enclosed from the Office of the Secretary of Defense. I had requested benefits for Marci from the Department of Health, Education and Welfare. My letter was forwarded to the DoD for reply.

My connection to HEW was Doctor MILLER at the U.S. Naval Hospital in Phila. [who] told me in 1968 Marci's defects were caused by my being poisoned by Dioxin (Agent Orange), sprayed in Vietnam. The DoD informs me that I was misinformed. They have no record of Dioxin causing deformities.

Marci was treated at the U.S. Naval Hospital in Bethesda, Md. for one year in 1968–1969. The Hospital staff wrote a Medical Journal about Marci. My wife and I signed release forms for the book and also authorized numerous photos to be taken of Marci, for placement in the book.

The Naval Department never allowed us to view the book. It is possible the book is about 245T with Dioxin contamination and related defects in children.

I can't accept the fact no one within our Government knows about the hazards of Dioxin poisoning. I learned from an article published by READER's DIGEST reporter John G. Fuller, during the 1976 Dioxin spill in Italy, the U.S. National Institute of Health and Stanford University used its most sophisticated equipment to isolate Dioxin in particles in animals, foods and soil samples removed from the scene.

A U.S. Department of Agriculture Specialist made the following recommendations to the Mayor of Seveso, Italy after the 1976 Dioxin spill:

1. Force the chemical Company involved to purchase land within specified zones.

2. Build a nine foot high plastic coated wire-mesh fence around the area.

3. Burn in an incinerator at 1000 degrees C all buildings, trees, asphalt road surfaces etc. in the contaminated zone.

Dr. Anne Walker, a dermatologist from Britain, who treated British workers for an earlier Dioxin spill informed Seveso officials the long-term effects of dioxin exposure may not surface until 10–15 years after exposure.

As I mentioned before, in 1968 Dr. MILLER at the Phila. U.S. Naval Hospital was the first to inform me of the hazards involved in contact with Agent Orange.

He stated he had encountered many still-born babies with massive deformities. Many other babies born only lived for a short period of time.

The doctor showed my wife and I a boy about the same age as Marci with no ears. The hospital hoped to either build ears for the boy or give him rubber ears. The doctor stated the boy was deformed as a result of his father's contact with defoliant spray in Vietnam.

I am saddened to know everyone has turned a blind eye to the veterans who stood up to be counted, when called to serve in Vietnam. Many of the vets need help now. A "few" like I have sick children requiring immediate attention. No one wants to get involved.

I stand alone in my struggle. I have all of the symptoms of the poison eating away at my guts. I burp 30–40 times per day, my kidneys hurt— I don't sleep well at night due to indigestion, I have a body rash and have recently learned that I have high blood pressure. I am 36 years of age.

It bothers me that we were not told by our superiors that Dioxin causes an off balance of body chromosomes and our off-spring could be born deformed.

I have not seen a doctor for my problems as I feel, after they get me, my days are limited. I do want to get Marci taken care of before I give in to the rot eating away within me.

I understand Senator Mark Hatfield of Oregon made the statement recently, "245-T (Agent Orange) is one-hundred times more lethal than nerve gas."

If you love your country as I do and I am sure you do, I feel you will open up the eyes of our people to this problem and see to it that our nation's heroes suffering from poisoning received in Vietnam are cared for.

> Sincerely,
> RONALD E. SMITH

Smith is not alone.

He is, in fact, on a long list that reads like a whispered roll-call from the Vietnam War. It is filled with as many as a million names—more, if you include the Vietnamese—but the numbers do not remain constant. Death, the Great Mathematician, regularly subtracts a lethal quota reserved in more ordinary times for men who already have experienced the joys associated with the prime of their lives.

It is a roster of dread in pursuit, from the sticky-sweet trembling in the pitch-black of a Southeast Asian jungle clearing to the shaded bulwarks of the purple mountains' majesty.

It is the shattered cry of Paul Reutershan, dead now, to his mother, "I got killed in Vietnam and didn't know it."

It is the deceit revealed in the shocked discovery made by Gilberto Reza, a Vietnam veteran too, and now a California congressional aide, that "the government and society have succeeded in making us politically and economically impotent, and now they want us eradicated from the social fabric."

It is the anxiety caused by periodic blind spells and permanent, acquired color blindness that makes John Woods, a strapping New York City bus driver, assert, "The VA refuses to admit the truth that they're wrong. To me it's a big cover-up."

And in a steaming wooden farmhouse in rural North Carolina, it is the indictment coerced from his rapidly waning strength, barely audible between chemically induced, lung-wracking wheezes, that rings out when Frank Moore, wounded at nineteen and dying at thirty-one, whispers, "I never missed combat. But all of a sudden they're punishing me, punishing me, punishing me. The government ain't intending it to be this way, I don't think."

No, Ronald Smith is not alone. Nor is his daughter Marci.

"Once you get into this and see what's involved," says Maureen Ryan, "the more you read, the more you realize it's the same symptomatology throughout the country. That's a lot of kids."

The symptoms, a veritable compendium of medical horrors, include nervous system disorders, especially the loss or decrease in sensitivity of the senses; numbness in the toes, fingers, legs and arms; painful and persistent boils and skin rashes, specifically chloracne, which impair normal functioning; psychological effects, including memory loss, confusion, depression and suicidal thoughts, uncharacteristic aggression or irritability, and blackouts; cancer, especially cancer of the liver; altered sex drive, including diminished interest or impotence in men and increased sexual activity in women; and a host of other characteristics ranging from nausea and dizziness to listlessness to extreme susceptibility to illnesses like the common cold and infections.

And that's only for adults.

Birth defects in children born to fathers exposed to Agent Orange include missing limbs, physical deformities, partially formed internal organs, spinal-cord growth outside the body, heart defects, psychological problems like hyperactivity and retardation, and frequently recurring sickness. Miscarriages and spontaneous abortions are also associated.

Maureen Ryan was not in Vietnam, but the war came crashing through her front door and into her home in Long Island nevertheless. It was brought back unknowingly and unwillingly by her husband Mike after thirteen months in the army.

Nor was Kerry Ryan in Vietnam, even though she bears the scars more vividly than a thousand four-star generals. Kerry, the Ryans' ten-year-old daughter born after Mike's return from overseas, came into this world with eighteen separate birth defects— among them twisted intestines, a hole in her heart, a deformed bladder and throat, missing bones, and deformed limbs. She also has no reproductive organs.

Mike, a sergeant on the Suffolk Country police force, connects Kerry's abnormalities to the drinking water in Vietnam. It was— probably still is—contaminated with Agent Orange.

"No one ever warned us about the hazards of the defoliant," he says.

Dioxin, the poisonous active ingredient in the herbicide Agent Orange, is called by scientists like the University of Wisconsin's Dr. James Allen, the acknowledged expert in the field, "the most toxic man-made substance known today." Between 1962 and 1970, it was sprayed by helicopters and C-123 cargo planes over more than 5 million acres of Vietnam, roughly 12 percent of that beleaguered country. Trucks and backpacks were also used to spread the substance.

The heaviest spraying, code-named "Operation Ranchhand" by LBJ's phrasemakers, occurred in the late 1960s when American troop strength was at its height. Most of the approximately 44 million pounds of the defoliant, containing 386 pounds of dioxin, was sprayed near U.S. base camps. A lot of it wound up in the ground and in drinking water. The winds, spreading it still farther, didn't know a Viet Cong from a Nebraska farmboy.

The purpose of all this activity was to remove the thick tree and foliage cover used by opposing soldiers and to destroy food crops in populated areas.

But the chemical, made by Dow, Monsanto, and three other companies, is so powerful it could, and did, knock down giant 150-foot hardwood trees in less than forty-eight hours. Areas sprayed with Agent Orange quickly became vast empty wastelands, where nothing moved, breathed, or lived. Dioxin is considered one hundred times more lethal than nerve gas (a favorite used in earlier wars). It is estimated that one medicine drop can kill twelve hundred people. A few ounces can wipe out the population of New York, if placed strategically.

In 1976, thousands of residents, including many workers, were contaminated with the poison after an accident at dioxin production facilities in Seveso, Italy. As a result, the Catholic Church and the Italian government both permitted abortions for all pregnant women who had been exposed. Many of those not having an abortion gave birth to babies with congenital defects.

Further, laboratory studies show that dioxin-infected animals develop cancer and other serious abnormalities. Other research and data point dramatically to a link between dioxin and a variety of diseases.

And as a legacy that will forever entwine the genetic destinies of two former enemies, symptoms among the Vietnamese in sprayed regions, especially among women and newborn children, are identical to those exhibited by Kerry Ryan, Marci Smith, and other American citizens. In 1970, in a fit of decency sparked by public outrage (and, probably, wartime strategic considerations), U.S. forces halted the spraying operations because of their effects on the population.

Somewhat incongruously, with a wave of bitter defiance, the outrage has been incorporated into the lexicon of at least one afflicted family.

"Last week, Jessie began a siege of 'Montagnard syndrome,' as I call it," reports Robin Lutz, the Brooklyn-born, part-Apache wife of a Vietnam veteran, referring to the hardy, independent Vietnam tribespeople who became burdened with Agent Orange poisoning. "She's got a hundred-and-four-degree fever, diarrhea, stomach cramps, and severe congestion. And all the medications are useless.

"All of my children have had that several times and I never knew what it was until I read about the Montagnards' children who developed it, and naturally it's dioxin-related." Robin's three children are constantly sick. In addition to Jessie, two-year-old Christine was born with a displaced hip and Jamie, three, has had thirty ear infections in two years. He may have a sensorimotor loss and is always taking medication. Jim and Robin Lutz spend sixty dollars a week on medical expenses. "I live at the doctor's," says Robin.

In 1979, the United States Environmental Protection Agency banned the domestic use of the herbicide containing dioxin. It was cancer-causing, the agency said. In Oregon, pregnant women seemed to have more miscarriages in an area that was heavily sprayed with the poison. Also in 1979, the manufacturers of the chemical filed a countersuit in federal court claiming, in essence, that dioxin has never been shown to cause any long-lasting ill effects, but if it does turn out to be harmful, the U.S. government is to blame because, the companies say, it was lax in warning users of its dangers.

Despite the evidence, and despite the torment, the VA is adamant in its refusal to acknowledge a service-connected relationship between Agent Orange and the statistically significant number of similar symptoms cropping up in veterans whose service records, not to mention their vivid personal recollections, show them to have been in sprayed areas, or who have handled or actually sprayed the chemical themselves.

The VA insists it needs "conclusive" evidence before it starts compensating dying veterans or their widows, even though Title 38 of the U.S. Code, the VA's legal authority, specifically instructs the agency to resolve any "reasonable doubt" in favor of the veteran. Apparently, increased liver cancer rates in an age group in which the fatal disease was heretofore virtually unknown is not reasonable doubt enough. Evidently, offspring with bodies broken and impaired in the same places and in the same way, produced by parents who shared the same preconditions, are not sufficient to sway the keepers of the wavering faith who look after the widow and the orphan.

Researchers have long known that correlations—that is, statistical associations—do not by themselves guarantee the existence of a cause-and-effect relationship. (Because the flag is run up the flagpole every morning it doesn't mean the sunrise is responsible, even though you can predict with a fair degree of accuracy the coincidence of both events.) Scientists, and VA administrators and statisticians, also know, however, that in the absence of a perfect universe, scientific certainty is often measured by degrees of approximations, not absolute answers. That's why, for example, surgeons discuss the probabilities, the risks, of success of an operation. Or why pharmaceutical suppliers hedge on the efficacy of a new drug. But surgeons still perform operations and pharmacies continue to dispense drugs.

The VA, however, still rejects Agent Orange disability claims despite a stronger statistical certainty—not to mention an overriding human tragedy—than that which existed when penicillin was first released to the public, or than that which predicted Three Mile Island would never pose a threat to human life.

What the VA is really saying is that *its* scientists see no connection, and that the veterans' data are just not proof beyond a reasonable doubt. What the VA is also saying is that money, squandered so freely to get the grunts over there to kill for America, is not available for those who have come home. Unlike used bullets, however, soldiers can get cancer.

The victims' fury at the VA's cautious inaction is palpable. Cleland, for instance, was confronted by angry Agent Orange vets and their families at a Senate hearing in California in early 1980.

Coming close to blows with some of them as he waited to speak, Cleland was taunted concerning his war injuries. "Did you lose your balls in Vietnam, too?" one vet asked.

Others ask the question differently.

"You're talking about millions of veterans who were in Vietnam itself. To provide compensation for these people is going to run into billions and billions of dollars, sure. I understand that. But for cryin' out loud, there is a problem, and it's gotta be looked at. Right?" Rocky Rocanelli is talking. He is sitting in the living room of his desert tract home in a growing suburb of Phoenix, the sun outside fading still another sclera of paint off the fins of the pre-gas-crisis vintage Cadillac waiting to be revitalized on the concrete driveway. A dartboard, filled to the bull's-eye with color-fully feathered steel pins, glares monocularly from the garage door onto the shimmers of dry heat making the neighbor's house undulate across the street.

Inside, where it is a little cooler, Rocky keeps the drapes drawn, not so much to keep out the heat as to deflect the light. Ever since he returned from Vietnam in the spring of 1969, the bright sunshine has bothered him. "I wake up invariably with these terrific headaches," he says, "just from the morning sunlight."

Something else happened to him since leaving twelve months of his life behind in the central highlands of South Vietnam, assembling bombs for the air force. In November 1971, Joan Rocanelli gave birth to a baby girl, their second child. Arlena was born with spina bifida (external spinal cord), hydrocephalus, dislocated hips, and clubbed feet. She has had fifteen separate surgical procedures.

"It took some time before we made the connection," Rocky recalls, "but when we did, we started putting two and two together and we realized that we had friends with children with such severe defects that some of them died. And all of us, the fathers anyway, were in Vietnam.

"This one friend, in Detroit, we didn't discuss it, but we knew there just gotta be a tie-in somewhere. That was always in the back of our mind."

Joan, like several of the other wives, also experienced a miscarriage.

"With all the same symptoms, it's not a coincidence. It can't be," Rocanelli insists. "I called my friend in Detroit, a while after his daughter died from the defects. I said, 'Kenny, I got some shit to lay on you you're not going to believe.' And I started telling him about Agent Orange. I was just hearing about it then. He said, 'Dammit! I knew it! I knew there was a link there somewhere.' "

Not according to the VA, there isn't.

"The VA is there, supposedly, to help veterans," Rocanelli, a New York transplant, continues. "I got brothers walking into the VA and they're telling 'em, 'Don't worry about it. It's nothing major. It's your nerves. You're upset.'

"Bullshit. Nerves does not cause cancer. Nerves does not cause chloracne. Nerves does not cause liver problems. It doesn't cause all these different symptoms. Look, it's a cover-up. There's no doubt about it. Most people would rather not deal with the Vietnam vet."

That includes the VA. Up until 1972, the VA provided employers with coded data that enabled them to weed out supposedly undesirable prospective employees. When a veteran walked in looking for a job, he was unaware that a certain series of numbers in a little box on his discharge papers—the so-called "Spin" designation, shorthand for Separation Program Number—revealed such things as the veteran's alleged attitudes toward authority, whether he had smoked marijuana while in the service, how reliable he was, or if he was obese. Unknown to the newly discharged vet, fired up with the enthusiasm of landing a job, the VA had provided the employer—usually the larger national corporations—with a sheet that deciphered the meaning of each of the numbers in the series. There were over five hundred categories in all.

Not infrequently, the Spin number was directly responsible for the veteran's continued unemployment—and the vet was never the wiser. In 1972, it was removed from all the records.

"It was a tremendous burden on the veteran," Rocanelli, now a Postal Service letter carrier, declares.

So was the fighting in Vietnam.

"The weapons that we had, the destruction that we caused, was unbelievable. Unreal. A lot of us who were in Vietnam would rather forget. We knew what was going on. What was the problem was that nobody *here* understood what was happening."

And, according to Rocanelli, they still don't.

"Like the Vietnam War, at least to me, the Veterans Administration is using a great cover-up. When you have all these problems placed right in front of your nose, the normal, semi-intelligent human being has to look at that, even if he's in the fifth grade, and say, 'Oh, shit. Something's going on.'

"The money's gotta be the reason. You're talking that you have to compensate these people for all the problems they went through. The VA doesn't want to have a line of people in their place that they have to take care of.

"First of all, they'd say, 'This guy's a Vietnam vet. Who the hell wants him anyway? Then we gotta take care of him. Ah, bullshit. Who wants to take care of this guy? Oh, my God. This one's got a kid that's got birth defects. We have to take care of them, too?'

"There's a lot of problems."

Recently obtained VA documents indicate the VA may well be aware of the problems, and their scope. However, the VA's response, outlined in the papers, has alarmed those involved in the fight for veterans' rights and lends substance to the charge by Rocanelli and others that a cover-up is in progress.

On September 3, 1975, the VA sent to the General Services Administration (GSA) a Request for Authority to Dispose of Records. The request covers "abstract card records [in the Tumor/Cancer Registry File] containing selected data for those patients admitted and treated for suspected or confirmed malignancies." The cards "contain detailed information regarding the type of neoplasm [cancer] . . . which is not in . . . the Patient Treatment File. Thus, these cards are not a duplicate of the computer file systems."

The document, approved a month later, authorizes destruction of the records of living patients after twenty years. The records of deceased patients "or patients lost to follow-up" can be destroyed after five years. Attached to the approved request are "Retention Limitations and Disposition" instructions to the Medical Administration Service, dated April 30, 1976, to "Destroy Immediately."

"What does this all mean?" Dr. Gilbert Bogen, a psychiatrist and former chief of staff forced out of his post at the North Chicago VA, writes in *Stars and Stripes.* "Is it possible that medical records belonging to Korean and Vietnam veterans have been destroyed? Are claims for service-connected malignancies being denied for lack of a medical record?"

The sense of urgency is not limited to Vietnam veterans whose claims of Agent Orange–induced cancer may be lost forever, and along with them any hope of establishing documented proof of its origins, by the hasty destruction of irreplaceable medical data. Another group with a vested interest is composed of the men exposed to large doses of radiation during experimental atomic bomb tests in the Pacific and the American West in the 1950s. Cancerous growths and other anomalies (some of them remarkably similar to those found in some of the Vietnam veterans) are now cropping up twenty to thirty years after the explosions—just the time frame within which the VA is legally permitted to destroy the only evidence of carcinogenic precursors the veteran may have.

Reason Warehime, a veteran of World War II and Korea from Riverdale, California, is one of them.

"In 1953 I was stationed at Fort Knox, Kentucky, and they come up one day and they said, 'Hey, Warehime. Do you want to be an observer out there at the Camp Desert Rocks with that atomic bomb deal?' And I said, 'Shoot, yeah, that sounds interesting.'

"Now, they said 'observer.' They didn't say 'guinea pig.' This is the part that burns me up about this whole deal, because now they're beating the guys who were made guinea pigs out of their deals, based on the fact that there were so many thousands of observers out there. But there is a definite difference between the guinea pigs and the observers."

Warehime, fifty-three, is a big, friendly, talkative man, almost bald except for close-cropped gray hair on the side of his head. He apologizes frequently for smoking his Carlton 100s. With a cigarette in his mouth, which is often, and his brown-tinted sunglasses set back on his nose, he looks strikingly like George C. Scott's version of General Patton.

Wounded "in more places than I can remember," Warehime wears a Stimtech electronic stimulator to prevent pain in his left leg and lower back. It is attached to a thick black belt with a silver buckle that is squeezed under a fair-sized belly.

His left leg is atrophied and looks as if it belongs to another person in comparison to his good right leg. Warehime is the chaplain at the Fresno VA and sports a brown pin on his blue sports shirt identifying him as a VA employee. The ID has a small cross on it. Lying on the desk in front of him is his medical chart. It is marked "confidential" because Warehime, who was very close to an atomic blast, has been exposed to radiation. Belatedly, 350,000 other GIs have realized the same thing: They were unwitting subjects in a massive experiment.

"It was in Nevada," he continues. "Out there where they were doing the bomb tests. Yucca Flats. They put me as first sergeant of about one hundred eighty-five officers. Then the day before the drop they come up and gave me a list. I wish I still had that. Oh, I'd give anything to still have that. They gave me a roster of two hundred fifty enlisted men. They said, 'These will be your men at the bomb drop tomorrow.'

"Well, it didn't dawn on me: Why aren't I going with my company of officers that are going out there as observers? So they take us out there and put me in this trench with two hundred fifty guys. They even told us we were two hundred fifty yards away from ground zero. It was a Hiroshima-size bomb. It was a tower shot. They had it on a five-hundred-foot tower to set it off.

"They had an airplane flying over with a chimpanzee in it. Remote control, to see what would happen. They had houses with mannikins in them. They had sheep. About a hundred yards in front of us they had a trench just like ours filled with sheep. To see, you know, what would happen.

"And then they set that durned thing off. There were no officers there. Of that roster of men, nobody knew the guy that was sitting alongside of him. They were all guys from different army bases all over the world that had been flown in there. No two men knew each other.

"Anyway, that darned thing went off. It was the first time I'd ever seen the bones in my hands that weren't on film. We had sunglasses on, with my hands over my eyes, and I could actually see the bones in my hands when that thing went off. In fact, I could see the outline of the guy sitting next to me. It was just like looking at an x-ray film.

"The lunch I put on the edge of the trench was all burned up. And the sheep, about one hundred fifty yards in front of us, they were barbecued. They hollered for us to get up and look at it. And we did. A ball of fire right over our heads. We were inside the stem. They told me to take the men in a skirmish line, march them down past where the tower was, to where the hole in the ground was down there and there would be trucks to pick us up.

"So I went down there. Sure enough, the trucks were there and they passed out a bunch of brooms. We didn't even have the radiation badges on . . . nothing. They told us to brush one another off with the brooms. Everybody kept telling us we had to be ten miles away from the thing.

"The thing that burns me up is now they're saying they put us in there to see what kind of fear response they got. They didn't get any fear response because we thought it was all approved and okayed. And we're infantry soldiers, combat men. We've been around artillery blasts before. That was no big deal. I mean, it was a big deal, considering it was one bomb, but we'd been around artillery barrages where the ground shook just as bad.

"Nobody's ever been closer than ten miles to that bomb. And the only thing I saved that even shows I was there—boy, if I only knew—was the Chamber of Commerce in Las Vegas passed out a cartoon diploma called the Order of the Droop to the guys that were at the atomic bomb blast, and that's the only thing I've got to prove that I was there."

The VA, of course, insists on more than that. As with the Vietnam vets, even though the symptoms among the atomic bomb vets are similar, benefits will not be paid. Not only has cause-and-effect not been established beyond a reasonable doubt, but in Warehime's case even his presence at the explosion is in question.

What happened after the blast is perfectly clear, however.

In 1954, about a year after his Yucca Flats experience, Warehime was sent to Germany.

"It was about six months after that that I started having trouble with my mouth," Warehime, who had a broken heel diagnosed by a VA physician as a sprained ankle, says, "Had toothaches all the time, and I had a full set of teeth. I couldn't eat nothing. I went to the dentist and he gave me medicine for pyorrhea and it didn't help. Finally, they pulled every daggone one of my teeth. All thirty-two of them at one smack, and all the nerves were exposed. The gums had receded back where all the nerves were."

Warehime also lost all his hair.

"But then it came back. Every bit of body hair I had disappeared. It came back real light and real thin. Crotch hair and everything. It was gone."

Warehime pauses in his long soliloquy, and digs out another Carlton.

"My wife and I had two children before I went to Korea," he finishes. "We had two boys and we wanted a girl. We never could have that girl. I was sterile ever since the bomb test. I've been tested. My wife's been tested. Nothing wrong with my kids. I keep telling the army this. I keep telling the VA this. They don't even pay attention. Not at all."

That refrain is now repeated by another generation of soldiers.

Agent Orange, so named because of the color of the identifying stripes on the container it came in, was only one of a number of differently hued herbicides used in Vietnam. Agent Blue, Agent Purple, and so on were also sprayed over a wide area of the country. But Agent Orange was the most toxic.

The association between the dioxin-contaminated Agent Orange and serious health disturbances like liver cancer and chloracne was in fact first noticed by a VA benefits employee in the Chicago regional office of the VA, Maude de Victor. She had never heard of Agent Orange when the wife of Charles Owen, a Vietnam veteran, called in 1977.

Owen was dying of cancer, Mrs. Owen told de Victor, and he blamed it on the herbicide. When Mrs. Owen called a second time after her husband's death and informed de Victor that the VA had refused her claim for survivor's benefits, the thirty-eight-year-old VA counselor began researching the spraying program. She located by January 1978 more than fifty cases similar to that of Charles Owen.

Hearing of her data collecting, Mrs. de Victor's VA supervisor ordered her to stop assembling the material. Maude de Victor took her statistics to Chicago's WBBM-TV, which aired an award-winning documentary, "Agent Orange, the Deadly Fog."

Even though the VA occasionally boasts that it was one of its own employees who first brought the effects of Agent Orange to public attention, the fact of the matter is that the reward for Maude de Victor's whistle-blowing was removal to a back office where her phone calls were screened, her job duties changed, and her contact with veterans restricted. Once, asked why she pursued the path she did, Maude de Victor answered, ignoring VA intimidation, "I have a commitment to the living, I have a commitment to the dead, and I have a commitment to the unborn."

Major lawsuits stemming from the use of Agent Orange have been filed by veterans hoping to reclaim damages. One of the court actions, in New York, is against the manufacturers of the chemical, contending they knowingly allowed dioxin to be used despite its harmful properties. Although the companies deny the charges, there is evidence that links dioxin with cancer and deformities.

One of the most alarming statements confirming the connection was an admission by the National Academy of Sciences, in a 1974 report cited in congressional testimony by Assistant Chief Medical Director Dr. Paul Haber in defense of the VA's efforts, that "the likelihood of long term, serious adverse health effects among persons other than the North Vietnamese or the South Vietnamese Montaignards is highly remote."

Commenting on the potential impact of the case, U.S. Judge George Pratt, ruling that the veterans' claims should be heard in federal court, said that "the estimated number of involved veterans ranges from thousands to millions and the estimated potential liability of the five [defendant companies] ranges from millions to billions of dollars." A similar suit, this one against the VA, was filed by the National Veterans Law Center in Washington, D.C., on behalf of seven individuals, the National Association of Concerned Veterans, Concerned American Veterans Against Toxins, and Agent Orange Victims International.

One member of Agent Orange Victims International is Rocky Rocanelli. He is, in fact, the group's Arizona director, and he feels very strongly about his victimization.

"A lot of my friends and myself have an aversion to hearing the 'Star-Spangled Banner' played anymore," he says a little self-consciously. Rocanelli, thirty-two, is heavyset and olive-skinned and likes Italian food. Like most Agent Orange victims, however, he must be careful with his alcohol, especially beer, because of the magnified effect it has on him.

"I know, that sounds disrespectful as hell. But if you turn around and just stop and look for a minute, what did the United States do for me? Besides take my ass over there, expose me to Agent Orange, let me have a birth-defected child, let me have the problems that I'm having and then say, 'I don't want to take care of you.'

"What we want is help. We are not asking for a lot. We're asking for what's due us. That's all. We were exposed to a herbicide which was very dangerous, that creates cancer, that creates birth-defected children, and somebody, somewhere along the line —whether it's Dow Chemical or the United States government— somebody is going to have to say, 'We screwed up. We're going to have to do something.'

"All right, I'm having a hard time making ends meet. But that's my problem, because I decided to let my daughter live. Big decision, right? But, if in fact Agent Orange did cause these problems, then, you know . . . I don't think it's fair for the insurance company to have to pay all the money they've been paying on her. And I don't think it's fair for me.

"Right now I'm angry. I'm angry that this happened. I'm angry that they're not looking at the problem, that they're ignoring the problem. I don't think you can ignore it much longer, because I got brothers out there that don't got the time. All those guys—we're going to have to have cancer checkups every year for the rest of our lives because we went over there and did something for our country. We still come back and get shit on. They don't want to give us the help. They don't even want to hear about us."

Right now, the most visible symptom for Rocanelli, aside from the light sensitivity, are the scars carried around by his daughter, a former March of Dimes poster child. But if his brothers, as he calls them, are suffering all around him, what does the future hold for him?

"You want an honest answer?" Rocanelli sighs. He pauses briefly, thoughtfully. He explains that, yes, at first the knowledge about the effects of Agent Orange did cause some tension, some anxiety. "I don't think about it," he blurts out, a little too fast. "I've got all these other brothers to think about right now."

Joan Rocanelli interrupts. "That's not true," she says quietly, looking at her husband. "I can tell when you're thinking about it."

Rocanelli sits back on the couch. "All right, well, yeah, sure, I think about it," he says. "Hey, I'd be asinine to say I don't think about it every now and then. I don't make it my main concern. My main concern right now is my daughter, my wife, my family." His voice drops. It is barely audible.

"And then comes my brothers out there who are really hurtin'." His voice rises, and then falls again. "And then I'll think about Rocky. When things slow down and there's nothin' happening," he says, his eyes far away, "I think about Rocky."

In 1979, finally responding to enormous pressure brought about by organized ad hoc veterans' groups, individual veterans, and some members of Congress, the VA convened an advisory committee to find the facts about Agent Orange. Typically, the VA started off on the wrong foot when it did not include a single Vietnam veteran on the committee. The reaction from the vets themselves was so vehement that Cleland agreed to add one veteran.

However, while veterans are dying from liver cancer at rates found only in elderly men, and women are continuing to have miscarriages, the advisory committee, composed of scientists and researchers, was given two years to come up with recommendations and a report. The group, obviously in no hurry to fulfill its mandate, meets once every three months. The air force, too, has agreed to investigate the matter. Its study is still bogged down in procedural concerns. For its part, the Department of Defense insists it just doesn't have the records that would pinpoint troop locations and sprayed areas during the war.

"From my perspective, I think the major area of difficulty here will be one of communication," Dr. James Crutcher, the former VA chief medical director who left office in late 1979 reportedly under a barrage of criticism from congressional committee members, staff and veteran groups alike, told the first gathering of the Agent Orange Advisory Committee. "Those of us in the biomedical field often say things and often our patients don't understand what we say, even though we think it is very simple. . . . Those patients of ours who are neither biomedical careerists or scientists, but perceive signs and symptoms as they affect them, and its possible relationship to long-term effects of herbicides, have their own language and their own mind-set."

Crutcher is right. It is hard to wade through all the hogwash. But he, and Cleland, and Haber, and the others, can clarify the situation with some simple words, a few strokes of the pen, and a bit of common decency. It is not the abused patients who are stuck in their mind-sets, as Crutcher puts it. It is the VA, with all its self-serving gobbledygook and ballyhooed pretensions, that is refusing to respond to an ever-increasing load of information, or to the cries for help from its fellow citizens.

If, indeed, Agent Orange is not the culprit, then what *is* causing the same symptoms in hundreds of thousands of men with shared backgrounds and experiences? Something happened to these veterans, and their families, in Vietnam—*something* is making them sick and die—and whether it was Agent Orange is almost irrelevant. The symptoms—the deaths, the defects, the distress—are all obviously service-connected. That is the bottom line. That is what matters. To say otherwise is un-American, inhumane, and, yes, a cover-up.

"The issue is humanity to man. And that's what's so shocking," says Joan McCarthy, the overwhelmed sympathetic ear to hundreds of vets at the Washington, D.C., office of Vietnam Veterans of America. McCarthy, swamped by orange folders whose over-flow covers two desks, works closely with veterans who have called in to relate their own particular story of VA unresponsive-ness. Veterans who complain of superficial and skeptical treat-ment by VA doctors supposedly obligated to examine carefully any veteran suspecting Agent Orange poisoning. VA hospitals that don't make their Agent Orange screening services known to the veteran population. VA hospitals, like the one at Northport, New York, whose "Herbicide Clinic" consists of one doctor—when he can be spared from his other, regular duties.

"What it boils down to is that these people are being treated like animals. Worse than animals. Some of the things are so horri-ble, nobody believes it. You can sit in front of a congressional committee and they say, 'Oh, come on.' Especially when you have a Vietnam veteran there who everybody thinks is crazy anyway."

The phone is constantly ringing for McCarthy, a former aide to two United States Congress members. The streaks of gray in her otherwise black hair belie the fact that she was only thirteen when the war was at its most ferocious in 1969. She is wise—and disappointed—beyond her years, and her phone bills at the office are enormous.

"Being from Harrisburg, I know how it feels," she says. "This whole Agent Orange thing is just like that—the way our govern-ment responds to people in general. The government has gone so far away from the people that I think we're headed towards a revolution."

"I feel that as a veteran, I'm entitled to decent care—everyone is entitled to decent care," says Michael Ryan, the cop from Long Island. "But it's not decent care at the VA. It's not even custodial care. The VA is almost bordering on the criminal."

"You know," says Maureen Ryan, "I played by the rules and got screwed. You feel like you've been insulted in a lot of different spheres. You feel you've been gang-raped. But you don't give up."

The Ryans, leaders in the lawsuit against the chemical compa-nies, have accumulated medical bills of over $75,000. "Once Agent Orange is cleaned up," Maureen says, "I want to see the VA cleaned up. I'll be damned if I'm going to let us send nineteen- and twenty-year-olds overseas again and when they return they're told, 'Well, we can't really help you—go take care of yourself and, maybe, if you don't really like it, go commit suicide.' It's a very sick system. It has to be cleaned up."

Ryan says she was never a crusading person. Not until Kerry came along.

"I want to be able to say to my daughter that when it [the Agent Orange situation] was discovered, the government rectified it. I would like to say that. Kerry is a dynamite kid, she really is. What they're taking away from her isn't fair. It just isn't fair."

And Robin Lutz, whose husband Jim has been showing increased signs of Agent Orange poisoning lately, has several bitter questions for Max Cleland and the VA. "Is my husband going to live to thirty-five?" she wants to know. "Is he going to live to forty?"

She doesn't expect a response soon.

"They don't care. It's good-bye, nice seeing you, boys. It's all money. But I'd rather have a healthy Jim than the money. What? Is the VA going to detoxify my husband? The SOBs are killing us. I can't take it anymore."

"Have you ever tried to waste yourself?" Frank McCarthy says into the white electronic box off to the side of his oval desk. It is 11:00 A.M. and already the glass ashtray is awash with Tareyton butts smoked down to the filter. Orange folders are everywhere. It is Frank McCarthy's thirty-fifth birthday and right now he is trying to save a man's life.

"That's why I was at Tampa," the voice comes back at him, a little gravelly through the telephone company's equipment. Still, the caller's emotions are clear. The marine at the other end has just spent three months at the Tampa VA for severe depression.

"How many times?" McCarthy asks.

"Just once."

The marine has called McCarthy (no relation to Joan) because he heard that Agent Orange Victims International (AOVI) was taking interviews over the phone, and that those doing the interviewing were, like those calling, Vietnam veterans who have experienced the pain.

AOVI, a national organization, was founded in 1978 by Paul Reutershan, a twenty-eight-year-old Vietnam veteran from Mohegan Lake, New York, who died of cancer that destroyed his abdomen, colon, and liver. On his deathbed, he told his mother that he now realized he had died in Vietnam, but never knew it. Frank McCarthy, currently president of the group, promised the dying Reutershan he would continue the fight to help Agent Orange victims throughout the world. In 1979, Australia, with the second largest foreign concentration of pro-American troops in Vietnam, launched its own investigation into the mysterious symptoms many of its former servicemen were beginning to display.

As McCarthy talks to the marine, he writes information on a lengthy, detailed form that will soon find its way into a fresh orange-colored folder: lumps on the body, unaccountable angry outbursts, two dozen jobs since leaving the service in 1968, depression.

"You have a lot of symptoms of Agent Orange dioxin process," McCarthy says into the air. It comes out into the marine's kitchen across the Hudson River in New Jersey. He suggests the marine go to the East Orange VA "and have them look at you."

The voice comes back across the river and out of the box with a hint of disbelief and disdain.

"They won't help me there," the marine says.

"We know it's bullshit," McCarthy says quietly, "but it will detect if you have liver damage."

The marine agrees, but only after McCarthy's urging.

"Call us if you need help, if you get depressed," McCarthy says before shutting off the box. "And if you get any flak at the hospital, call me."

The marine doesn't seem to want to let go of a friendly voice, a comforting moment. Before he hangs up, he tells McCarthy of his four-year-old daughter who died of some kind of blood disease. The doctors were never quite able to diagnose what it was.

"I've been married nine years," the Vietnam veteran says haltingly. The static from the box is unable to conceal the tears in his throat. "She's a good woman."

McCarthy blinks away from the receiver. "All our women are good, putting up with our bullshit," McCarthy says barely audibly.

McCarthy turns back to the work of the day. In his lapel is a First Division army pin. On his desk, poking out from the clutter, is a small American flag stuck in a red plastic holder. The wall behind him is filled with pictures. Of McCarthy in Vietnam. Of a plane spewing a white plume of herbicide, with the caption, "Only we can prevent a forest." Of a color photo of McCarthy shaking hands with Jimmy Carter at a White House reception for veterans just minutes before he loudly interrupted the president's remarks to plead for help for Agent Orange victims.

There is also his Purple Heart certificate and, laminated and framed, the document he received for his Bronze Star.

Almost obscured by all this is a small round red and blue cloth patch. It is inscribed: "Vietnam Veteran and Proud."

McCarthy runs the office in New York with the monies he gets from his own disability compensation benefits, as do other AOVI vets around the country who run regional offices. Frank McCarthy is one of those people—like Bobby Muller, like Dave Christian, like Rocky Rocanelli—who has seen the war and transcended its meanness to make his life a resource for others. One of the traits that marks them is the ability to put their compassion and concern into a tangible perspective.

"If you look back into history, you'll see that the World War II vets were treated badly, the World War I vets were treated badly. The Korean War vets were forgotten totally. It happens in every war. The veterans who fought the war, when they come back, they're forgotten.

"The difference between us and the World War II vets—they were treated just as badly as we were—is that they came back en masse. Millions of people. They got treated badly but they all came together and joined those organizations. They lobbied and they got good benefits programs. The thing with us—we came back one at a time. We were snatched out of society, put into a war situation alone, snatched out alone, and brought back into a society alone that was apathetic to our needs, that wanted to forget the Vietnam War.

"We got the brunt of the worst of the war. We got the stigma of being undesirables, of being William Calleys who ran around killing women and children. We got treated like criminals, instead of like heroes, which we were."

The VA, for one, certainly did not treat McCarthy as a hero.

"It's a long, drawn-out story," he starts hesitantly. "I got shot up and blown up and got shrapnel in vital areas of my body. And I get pain every day. We were ambushed by a company of VC. We were a recon platoon. So we fought 'em off and I got shot up."

He is chillingly unemotional in the retelling.

"After coming back to the States is when all the problems started. I got discharged and I was in a lot of pain. I still am in a lot of pain. I never asked anything from the government except what I was supposed to get, and that's medical benefits and an education. I tried to get medical treatment in Newark [at the VA] and I got treated like a piece of shit, so I just left and said the hell with it, I don't need this.

"I came back to the States and tried to use my educational benefits and went six months without a check. Got evicted from my apartment. Got a piece of shrapnel coming out of my penis, blood all over my pants, and I go to the VA to get my money so that I don't get evicted and they send me to a mission in the Bowery with derelicts.

"That's where they send the vets. And here I got blood all over my pants and my brains are pounding out of my head, I'm a physical and psychological wreck and they send me to the Bowery and the derelicts.

"So I said from that point on I was going to get every benefit I had coming or they're going to kill me. Either I'm going to get it or they're going to kill me, one or the other. So I got one hundred percent disability, and I fought to get it—congressional hearing through [former Senator Jacob] Javits's office and I went through the whole fight. I'd go down there and turn over a desk and scream and holler. That was the way it had to be done."

In 1965, Frank McCarthy was in one of the first combat units to go to Vietnam. He says the experience—he was point man for his platoon, perhaps the most hazardous job on the ground—made him sick to his stomach, and forever changed his perception of his country. Filled with the legacy of President Kennedy, McCarthy was abruptly cut short when he realized "the politicians were running the war, and we weren't allowed to fight. They should have pulled us out in '65. I found out the reasons why they didn't one Sunday morning when I went downstairs and bought a New York *Times* and brought it back up and opened it up and there were the Pentagon Papers. And I got physically ill. I threw up. I had a blinding headache the rest of the day. It really destroyed me, because it showed that we weren't in Vietnam to stop communism, we were in Vietnam to generate capital for the corporations.

"And later on, we found out about Agent Orange."

McCarthy doesn't like to talk about himself. "You have to realize that I'm representing thousands of veterans with the same problems," he says by way of explanation. "So, I'm coming from a position the same as them. Their stories are important, too."

In fact, McCarthy and his organization have documented more than 7,500 of those stories, working out of his apartment in Manhattan. With his curly hair, dark skin, and Mediterranean nose, McCarthy looks 100 percent Philadelphia Italian. His name gives him away.

Pressed, he talks some more of his own experiences.

"I've had no treatment. None. It's a whole catch-twenty-two. I've gone to the VA. They sent me for psychological counseling. One doctor sat there and said, 'Well, clearly that shrapnel in your penis shouldn't be bothering you, you've had it so long, so the pain is psychological. So we feel that if we operate and take that shrapnel out of your penis, then your mind will say it's not in there so you won't get the pain anymore.' And he's very nervous, and he's saying, 'I'll operate on you and we'll take it *right* outta there and everything will be okay with you.' And I looked at him and I says, 'You're gonna operate on me down there? You're fuckin' crazy. I'll never let a maniac like you . . . You can't even light your fuckin' cigarette. And you're gonna cut on me down there? Forget it.'"

McCarthy tried Walter Reed next. "The VA said I couldn't go there because it's only for people on active duty. I'd have to join the army, unless I was a congressman or a senator or the president. So that's the catch-twenty-two. How many civilian doctors know how to deal with a guy who's got shrapnel in his prick?

"The reality is, I went four years where I couldn't fuck at all because of the shrapnel in my penis. I still got shrapnel in my penis, I still got pain. I tried to commit suicide just like Charlie, the guy who just called, because when you can't make love, you're not a man at all. You're nuthin'.

"And when you go to the VA and they tell you it's all in your mind, you don't give a shit whether it's in your mind or whether it's in your body. You just got it. And . . . nuthin'. There's no reason for you to live. Life is absolutely horrible.

"I tried [suicide] three times, the last time in '74. In '75 I finally won my victory against the VA.

"So, I have my problems, too, and that's what kinda keeps me in the fight. I'm fighting not only for thousands of other veterans, but for myself as well. We are the victims. We come totally from the position of the victims. Granted, not all eight thousand [who have called AOVI] are Agent Orange victims, but they're all suffering from one thing or another, which all gets back to the same thing—criminal neglect."

The morning sun is beginning to surmount the nearby skyscrapers, and sporadic slivers of light are falling on the little backyard sitting area visible beyond the oval desk through the sliding glass doors. From a short distance, the soft island seems lost in the sea of harshness.

McCarthy, his tan slacks and brown shirt freshly laundered, leans back against the file behind him. It is labeled "Data on Vietnam Era Veterans." He would rather talk about them, their suffering, their steadfastness in the onrush of adversity, their aching appeals to the VA and to reason, to their government, for help and understanding.

Vietnam is out of the file cabinet now. Vietnam is all over the United States, in its towns, its slums, its rivers and factories, its hospitals. It is interwoven into the fabric of America, indeed, into the very genetic structure of the nation.

McCarthy lights another Tareyton, and speaks of others. Leaving the talk of himself, his animation returns in a flood.

"The birth defects are the major portion of our thrust against the chemical companies, against the VA," he says, "because we're sick of medical studies and scientific studies and surveys, and scientists and doctors. We're sick to death of them.

"They're all fighting it and meanwhile we are the victims, again. To us, we'll never be able to prove that Agent Orange causes cancer. We're not going to win for the suicides, we're not going to win for the psychological aspects, the liver damage.

"The only way we're going to beat the VA and beat the chemical companies is through our children. Because the birth defects on our children have never been seen in medical science before *except* in animal experiments with dioxin. That's all the proof we need. We don't want any more proof. We don't give a shit anymore. We're sick to death of it. I'm sick of goin' on television shows with VA guys and they sit there and say, 'We don't have proof.' The proof is in our children. They can say it's a Vietnam vets issue, but it isn't. It isn't. It's a humanitarian issue."

With human statistics: In twelve years of combat, 57,000 soldiers were killed as a result of the war. Between 1974 and 1980, over 51,000 vets have died in the United States, with 5,000 cancer deaths among them. *Veterans are dying at almost twice the rate of death in actual combat.* The American government—American biochemical technology—is killing American soldiers faster and more economically than the Vietnamese enemy did.

"The VA is inept, inefficient, and should be phased out—it does not work," McCarthy says flatly.

Then, anguished and determined, he picks up the ringing white phone at his elbow. "We don't want to exist as an organization, but we have to," he says before punching the "talk" button. "The VA just isn't doing its job. We have to exist.

"It's already too fuckin' late for too many guys."

Over the box, a frightened veteran, speaking slowly and deliberately, starts to tell Frank McCarthy about these painful red blotches all over his skin . . . .

McCarthy pulls out another fresh orange folder, and starts writing.

7

8IO VERMONT AVENUE, N.W.

The most telling thing about Max Cleland is this exchange
with free-lance writer Tracy Kidder, reported in *The Atlantic* of
March 1978. Kidder, a Vietnam veteran himself, had just finished
describing Cleland's warm personal relationship with President
Carter. He pointed out that Cleland was the first Vietnam veteran
to head the VA. (At thirty-four, Cleland was also the youngest.)

Kidder: "Quite a success story."

Cleland, beaming: "Or else a very revealing study of political
ambition."

Kidder: "Cleland enjoys talking about his political ambitions.
He has said that he would like to be governor of Georgia and he
has been known to gaze out the window above his desk, across
Lafayette Park toward the White House, and say, 'Anything's possible.' "

The second most telling thing about Max Cleland is this quote
from an interview in his tenth-floor office suite late one Wednes-
day afternoon in August 1979.

Cleland, with a salary of $57,500, is eagerly discussing his active public relations effort to improve the attitude of VA employees toward the veterans they are hired to serve. "If you establish a behavior system whereby good attitudes pay off, then you've got the current flowing in your direction."

He offers as an example a woman employee in Los Angeles who, over the telephone, saved a veteran from committing suicide.

"This year in our 'VA—May I Help You?' campaign, we're tying money to compassion and sensitivity," Cleland says. "I am writing a personal note to her, and I am going to make sure that she gets a financial reward for that compassion and sensitivity. I've already made some twenty-dollar and thirty-dollar awards right on the spot. You know, individual action, boom, you get an individual reward.

"I have opened the system up, and I went on a hotline to one hundred seventy-two hospitals and also to the regional offices, and I said this is the way we're doing it. We're not only into the compassion and sensitivity thing, we're now putting money behind it."

He does not acknowledge the irony.

"That little nursing assistant out there," he continues, "when she finds that her friend, who is also a nursing assistant on the next ward, got twenty-five dollars for helping that guy up out of bed over there when he couldn't find anybody, and she went the extra mile or she stayed an hour after work, or whatever, then at that level it's going to start making a difference.

"What I'm trying to show you is that we have actually got a game plan to attack the question of compassion and sensitivity, because you've got to work at it as a management problem, which it really is.

"And you've got to work at it every day, every year."

The third most telling thing may only be a reflection of his presidential mentor's capacity for confusing loyalty with competence, but it is informative nonetheless. Acknowledging that she is not a veteran, nor has she had any VA experience "before Max asked me to help him out," Marthena Cowart, Cleland's staff assistant and fellow Georgian, drawls, "I'm as wide-eyed as you are about this."

Cowart is extremely protective of Cleland. She does her best to curtail the length of the interviews he gives, for example, and seems especially put-upon when the conversation turns to unpleasant matters. To Cleland's credit, he generally pays her no mind. But Cowart, who actually functions as media guide and conduit to her boss, became particularly agitated when one recent interview focused on the subject of Cleland's war injuries.

The official VA press handouts and the presumptuous "Suggested Introduction of Max Cleland, Administrator of Veterans Affairs" simply state that his wounds—the severing of both legs and his right forearm—were the result of a grenade explosion east of Khe Sanh, Vietnam, in April 1968, four weeks before he was scheduled to go home. He was a captain in the First Air Cavalry Division at the time, a battalion signal officer responsible for radio communications. He is now a triple amputee.

But the fact that he didn't receive a Purple Heart—unusual in a war that saw them dispensed like candy—has raised some speculation about the incident. (Purple Hearts are awarded to fighting personnel wounded in combat or in a combat zone.)

There are some who suggest that Max Cleland's war wounds were the result of a fragging: purposely harmed—usually with the intent to kill—by his own men for personal reasons. It was often directed toward officers in the field who were seen as recklessly risking their men's lives. It was not an uncommon occurrence in a war that had many uncommon occurrences. The military doesn't like to talk about fraggings. "There was a large incidence of that going on in the Signal Corps office overseas," says Dave Christian, like Cleland a decorated captain. Christian doesn't go beyond that except to say he has heard "speculation" about Cleland's injuries.

"There's been some general gossip that he was playing a game of 'hot potato' with a grenade, and it went off," says an older veteran, a former top-ranking national service officer and longtime congressional aide.

"But I don't know. I really don't know."

The issue is pertinent because it reflects directly on the leadership abilities of a man charged with overseeing a large and influential governmental agency where the chain of command and respect for authority are almost as ingrained as in the military itself. And it also reflects on the perceived abilities of a man who has sought high state office (he was a Georgia state legislator for two terms in the early seventies, when he met Carter, and lost a bid for lieutenant governor in 1974) and who speaks openly of pursuing political office again in the future.

Further, if the rumors are just that, rumors, the fact that suspicions have been raised at all speaks volumes about the way a man is seen by the men and women he expects to lead.

"If Cleland acted in Vietnam the way he's acting as administrator today, then the probability of his being fragged is great," says Forrest Lindley, Jr., a former Green Beret combat captain who spent almost two years in Vietnam and who more recently has helped write congressional legislation for veterans. "He would never have been able to get away, in Vietnam, with putting his interests and his superiors' interests above the welfare of his troops," adds Lindley, who knows Cleland and finds him to be a "political" person who is "sincere, in his own way."

"Every story I've heard, and having spent twenty months in Vietnam and being a combat officer, certainly leaves that [fragging] possibility open."

During a two-hour interview with Cleland in August 1979, I asked him if he had been fragged. Cowart, who was already trying to get the session ended, immediately asked, angrily, who would say a thing like that. She was visibly shaken.

Cleland, with measured equanimity, didn't hesitate to reply.

"Oh, no, I wasn't fragged. I wasn't fragged," he said. "It was a friendly grenade. I mean, it was a secure LZ [landing zone] in the operation at Khe Sanh. I got off a chopper with a radio team of two people, and we had a couple of radios, and I was the last one off the chopper. And I turned around to look at the chopper take off, and when the chopper took off I looked down at the ground and there was a grenade.

"Well, you know, we all had grenades dripping off of us. I had them strapped onto me, too, onto my flak jacket. And, quite frankly, I thought it was one of my grenades that had dropped off. Well, what apparently had happened was that when I jumped off the chopper, the thing had fell [*sic*] off my flak jacket and the pin had come out, so when I reached down to get it . . .

"I don't really know where it came from, but I was the last guy off the chopper, and when the chopper took off, I ran under the blades, right? I ran out from the base of the chopper, ran under the blades, turned around, and watched the chopper take off. And there it was on the ground. I've thought about it a lot. I think it probably dropped off my own pack and when I reached down to get it, I wasn't able to touch it because it exploded just before I reached it.

"So, the two guys who were with me had the radios and the generator, and they were already going the other way to set up the radio relay operation on this hill. So, in effect, I was the only guy within about ten meters of the thing. I went back to where the chopper had been, back to the grenade, reached down to get it, and it exploded.

"So, I wasn't fragged and I wasn't playing around with it, you know. It was just one of those freak accidents of war, and the reason I was not entitled to a Purple Heart was because it was apparently a friendly grenade on a friendly LZ. We weren't under attack. We weren't under fire. It was just one of those freak accidents of war. You know, in effect, these things happen. These things occur."

Cleland's reported accounts tend to vary.

In a February 21, 1977, interview in the Washington *Star,* just four days before his Senate confirmation hearings, Cleland told reporter Judy Flander, "It [the grenade] must have dropped off somebody's pack. People were milling around near it. Nobody else realized it was there, much less that it was live. My reactions were reflexive—to investigate, to get the thing out of the way."

Flander reports that his battalion was *loading* the chopper when Cleland noticed the grenade.

The incident, which eventually landed him in VA treatment and then a wheelchair, takes another twist in Myra MacPherson's

April 18, 1977, Washington *Post* story—two months after the Senate hearings and seven weeks after Cleland took office—where MacPherson points out that Cleland has been called a hero for having saved the lives of others around him when the grenade exploded. (Cleland himself, a Bronze and Silver Star recipient, always vigorously denies the hero characterization.)

"Cleland," MacPherson reports, "says his shielding others from the blast was only reflex action to a 'freaky war accident.' A live grenade *rolled off a supply truck* and Cleland moved toward it to throw it away. (Italics added.)

" 'I never touched it. The explosion blew me backwards . . .'" Cleland told MacPherson.

Viet vet Tracy Kidder, recounting the jumping-off-the-chopper theory, concludes cryptically in *The Atlantic,* "It is not known how the grenade came to be there or who had pulled the pin and why, but Cleland assumed it wasn't live."

Whichever account is the more plausible—falling off a flak jacket or rolling off a truck; tossing it away from milling soldiers or retrieving it with no one around—it is hard to understand how the grenade could have been activated in the first place. To remove the pin from the device, which arms the weapon, the pin is slipped through a small hole in the grenade, thereby priming it to be exploded. However, in order to actually trigger the weapon, another piece of metal, called a spoon because of its shape, has to be released. On release, the spoon makes a loud popping noise and flies off into the air. Within five seconds, the grenade explodes.

Veterans experienced with the hand grenades used in Vietnam point out that it is virtually impossible for a grenade to become "live" after simply falling off a truck or a flak vest. There is just no way there would be enough force to get the pin through the restraining hole, they say, without the effort a human hand, adrenaline running, would exert.

Still, if Cleland's present version is correct, he should have heard and/or seen the spoon go flying. Even if he hadn't, its absence from the weapon on the ground should have told him beyond any doubt that it was alive, and he should get the hell away. It is curious, too, that, since no one was in the area risking injury or death if it did explode, why Cleland didn't do the sensible thing —get as far away as possible as fast as possible. Then, if the thing hadn't exploded by the count of five, he could go back and get it, taking as much time as he wished.

As he himself said, he was approximately ten meters (more than thirty feet) from the grenade when he noticed it. Several seconds, by then, had already ticked off. Indeed, he hardly had time to reach it before it exploded.

"The killing radius is five meters [about fifteen feet]. That's when you're a dead person," explains a former combat marine who spent most of his time in Vietnam in I-corps. "But the wounding radius is fifteen meters [forty-five feet]."

If Cleland was right in his estimate of ten meters distance from the grenade, then he was virtually assured of "only" an injury if he just stayed where he was. And there was no compelling reason for him to retrieve the hand grenade. All he needed to do was wait five seconds.

"The first thing you learn," says the marine, "is get down. His actions don't make sense to me."

According to one of Cleland's top assistants, Dean Phillips, himself a decorated combat veteran, Cleland was not fragged. Phillips says he asked Dick Sweet, Cleland's commanding officer and now a high-ranking VA official, about the possibility. "Max was a communications officer who didn't know about grenades," Phillips says. "Shit, he didn't know a grenade from a muffled fart. It was stupid. He just had no experience with grenades, like most people in the rear."

Phillips also recalls talking with Cleland in an informal social setting before he was named VA administrator. Cleland, he notes, volunteered for Vietnam after tiring of his position as aide-de-camp to the commanding general of the Army Signal Center and School in Fort Monmouth, New Jersey.

"I'm no hero," Cleland reportedly told Phillips.

"It was a trick of fate," suggests Al Zimmerman, a Korean War combat medic and first sergeant at Walter Reed hospital in Washington, D.C., where Cleland first recuperated. "The grenade was pulled off his bandolier, and it was live once the pin was pulled.

He tried to throw it away from the crowd. I remember it because it was so unusual."

Still, the questions linger.

"A lot of asshole things happened over there," says Ron Robertson, a Special Forces instructor for five years and an expert on weapons technology. "I'm not saying how it happened, but if it did happen the way Cleland describes it, it would be a freak accident.

"Those things just don't happen like that."

The Veterans Administration central office in the nation's capital occupies an eleven-story wedge-shaped gray government building across H Street from Lafayette Park and an imposing statue of Gen. Thaddeus Kosciuszko, Son of Poland.

Inside the small but busy lobby, the visitor's attention is caught by a small color photo of Max Cleland, hanging between a bank of elevators and the information desk. On the desk is the notice "Welcome," poised over the VA logo in red, white, and blue. A brown and white sign stands next to the ground floor Veterans Benefits Assistance office. It reads, "Government ID Required— Visitors Register at Desk."

Standing near a brief history of VA benefits programs, L. Dunklin is keeping tabs on things. He is dressed in blue and he is wearing a cap on his head. On his shirt it says, "Halifax Security Guard." Armed, he also carries his billy club as he watches everyone who comes and goes, including those pushing a wheelchair through the automatic front doors.

On the tenth floor, double glass doors with "Administrator of Veterans Affairs" painted above them separate Cleland and his staff from the rest of the building. Rumor has it that the doors, which can be locked, were installed a number of years ago after a previous administrator was briefly held hostage in his office by some disgruntled vets seeking redress.

The main reception office in Cleland's suite in room 1006, however, is wide open. Across the parquet floor, a window overlooks the White House a couple of blocks away.

Dominating the room is a very stark four-foot-by-eight-foot black Plexiglas wall hanging. Flanked by full-size American and

VA flags in staffs, the bold white letters spell out the VA motto—
"To care for him who shall have borne the battle, and for his
widow, and his orphan." The passage is excerpted from a section
of Lincoln's Second Inaugural Address.

With malice toward none; with charity for all; with firmness in the right,
as God gives us to see the right, let us strive on to finish the work we are
in; to bind up the nation's wounds, to care for him who shall have borne
the battle, and for his widow, and his orphan—to do all which may
achieve and cherish a just and lasting peace among ourselves, and with
all nations.

"You have to realize," Cleland says as he munches on some
crackers resting on the six-foot round wooden table set at one end
of his spacious corner office, "that part of the game here in Washington, in any group, whether it's veterans' organizations or labor
unions or whatever, is that they're in the business of advocating.
And more and more is never enough.

"Part of it you have to discount as rhetoric. What I try to do is
separate the rhetoric from the real concerns. I think there are
some real concerns. I don't have any doubt about that."

Cleland loves to talk. He has, in fact, learned to take a natural
inclination and turn it into a political asset. He will answer your
questions before you ask them, preferring, and frequently suc-
ceeding in the attempt, to go off in his own direction. As a result,
he comes off as subtly evasive. Pinning him down verbally is a
challenge, but once a direct question is allowed to slip through his
self-selected barrage, he will respond in a paragraph or so, then
take off again.

Every comment is enthusiastically, cheerfully offered. He
speaks, if any soft-drawling Georgian can be said to so speak, in
spurts of boyish exclamation points. His youthful features reflect
this energy.

Once a husky athlete—he still keeps a basketball on the bottom
shelf of his office, occasionally tossing it into a makeshift basket
—he is now heavyset, tending to flab, almost baby fat. His reddish
sandy hair, although beginning to thin, is usually associated with
a younger man. The stub of his right arm, used in conversation

for emphasis and expression, is as active as his good left arm. On his tan short-sleeve shirt is pinned a "VA—May I Help You?" button.

Perhaps the most significant part of Max Cleland's physical presence is his attitude toward his disability. He makes a point of greeting and saying good-bye to visitors at his office doorway, like any good executive. Offering his left hand for a handshake, Cleland then accompanies, via his black wheelchair, the guest into the office. As the conversation proceeds, you suddenly realize that he is no longer in the wheelchair but is, instead, sitting quite comfortably in a regular blue chair, color coordinated with the couches and wallpaper.

The switch has been made with such smoothness, with so little effort, that you can't remember his doing it. The same is true when Cleland reverses the process as he ushers his guest to the door.

Although he is quick to point out that his own experiences as a patient in the VA in the late sixties were not good—"They treated me like a number," he says—and that he will be a VA consumer "until the day I die," it is hard to escape wondering how his own healthy recovery may be influencing his attitudes toward those veterans who are still significantly dependent on the VA, and other agencies, for assistance.

"A lot of people are in it to throw rocks," he continues. "It's a focus on the political—what looks to them to be the key issues, but which to me are issues which more appropriately fill the editorial pages than the fact pages."

He suggests that some of the more important needs don't have a constituency to push for them. And he resents not getting credit for creating that constituency.

"One of the real horrors I found on coming here was that, number one, in the largest rehabilitation system in the country, centrally directed, there was not even a chief of Physical Therapy! And there are nine hundred physical therapists out there! There was not even a head of Rehabilitation Medical Services, and there was nobody to pull rehabilitation services together in the Department of Medicine and Surgery!

"If I had been in one of the service organizations, I'd have been screaming bloody murder about that for years. But that was not one of their interests. I don't know why. It's one of mine."

As a result, Cleland appointed a Vietnam veteran to head up the Rehabilitation Medical Service, he named a chief of Physical Therapy, and he appointed a blind Korean veteran to run the blind rehab service. He also has upgraded and expanded alcoholism treatment programs, although one of his biggest embarrassments was his heavily publicized visit to the San Francisco alcohol treatment unit early in his tenure. To his dismay, Cleland learned upon his arrival that there was no such program. "Sixty Minutes" duly informed the American public about it.

Cleland did fire the unit's head and transferred the hospital director. "It's a very fine operation now," he notes.

"I've spent a lot of time and a lot of effort on upgrading alcoholism services in the VA," he says somewhat bitterly, "but there is not a constituency beating on my door to upgrade the services. I don't get any thanks at all.

"But alcoholism is the single greatest diagnosis the VA health-care system has. It's not cancer, it's not lung disease, it's not flat feet, it's not the flu. It's not any one of those things. And it's not war-related disease or disability. It's not gunshot wounds, it's not spinal-cord injury. It's not amputations. It's alcohol. And until 1970, the VA didn't even have one alcohol treatment unit. Since I've been here, we've added thirty-five alcohol treatment units to the Veterans Administration, but do I get thanks for that?

"And yet, alcoholism is the greatest single drug problem among Vietnam veterans. But there is not a constituency for that out there. You know what the constituency focuses on? It focuses on whether I go to the White House and burn my wheelchair on the White House lawn in a big display of fighting for veterans.

"Sure, they think if I don't go over there and do that, somehow I'm not doing my job. They somehow choose to selectively ignore a lot of the basic accomplishments that I have been able to make in the last two years." Among them, Cleland lists the hiring of some twenty-five thousand Vietnam veterans in the first two years of his office, raising them to 16.3 percent of all VA employees by the end of 1978. Six percent of the total number are disabled.

Cleland is especially proud of the establishment of the VA's readjustment counseling program for Vietnam-era veterans. Ever the PR-sensitive administrator, Cleland labeled the effort, which officially began October 1, 1979, "Operation Coming Home."

Ironically, it is widely acknowledged as the VA's most visible and damning reminder of its abysmal failure to respond satisfactorily to its youngest generation of fighting men and women. But Cleland, in part correctly, hails it as a triumph.

For more than ten years, VA staffers have suggested that returning Vietnam veterans were not having their needs met by traditional VA services. The veterans themselves quickly learned to stay away from the system that, as it did Cleland, treated them impersonally.

As far back as 1971, then-Administrator of Veterans Affairs Donald Johnson told a series of VA-sponsored, countrywide seminars that surveys conducted several years earlier by his agency "indicated that these [Vietnam] veterans were different in many respects and that if we were to meet their needs, basic changes in VA methods and operations were essential."

In 1979, Congress was finally convinced to go along with the idea that a separate program, serving Vietnam vets, was needed. Although the Senate consistently passed appropriate legislation over those years, the House balked until President Carter and Cleland, urged on by a vocal constituency, persuaded the legislators to pass the Veterans Health Care Amendments Act of 1979.

Previous VA administrators, despite all their surveys, were lukewarm to the proposal.

"Why didn't it pass earlier?" Cleland asks, not without anger. "Because the president was against it in '70, '71, '72, '73, '74. And the Veterans Administration took a positive role against it. Senator Cranston, when I testified, said that for the first time in five years the VA had come out a friend of psychological readjustment counseling.

"You think there would have been a prayer if President Carter wasn't for it, if I didn't fight for it? Where's the thanks for that?"

Cleland's victory, late as it is, is somewhat historic. Cleland did have to battle entrenched interests who preferred to spend the money elsewhere. The response was not unlike that afforded the World War II Bataan veterans who more than thirty years ago waged a fight to convince a reluctant government that forty-two months in a Japanese concentration camp might cause disabilities and problems that would surface only after many years. As recently as ten years ago, some of these veterans, with eye problems and psychiatric difficulties, encountered resistance when they sought out treatment for what they considered were service-connected disabilities.

Now, Vietnam veterans are finding a similar response. Sometimes it even comes from surprising quarters.

"I really don't think the VA has to develop anything new. We just need to let people know what we have," says Richard Olson. Olson is a navy veteran who was hit three times in three weeks and spent a year in the hospital from wounds suffered while on duty in Vietnam. Olson is also chief of Program Development for the VA's Mental Health and Behavioral Sciences Services. He disagrees strongly with his former comrades-in-arms.

"There are a lot of people in the VA who care," he says. "I get a little confused sometimes, where all this bad press comes from. I've never had my checks come late, I've never had any problems with the VA, so it's hard for me to understand the problems of a lot of guys. I just didn't have them."

Olson, who has a master's degree in hospital administration, says he was helped tremendously by the interest of a VA counselor "who took me by the hand and showed me how to go about getting the benefits. He said if I wanted to help the cause of peace, that sort of thing, I should make use of as many VA benefits as I could. He told me, 'If the VA pays every veteran what they'll pay you, they won't be able to afford another war.' "

Olson has little tolerance for the veteran who complains of the Vietnam veterans' high unemployment rate, or the psychological problems they brought home with them—areas of concern that Cleland's new psychological readjustment program is specifically mandated to address. "Sometimes I have to bite my tongue around here. All you hear is, the poor Vietnam veteran, shat on, not cared for, all of that. I don't believe that. When you come right down to it, it was all there for the asking. You might have to look for it. It's a struggle. But it's there."

"It's not true that the Vietnam veteran has been treated unfairly," says Thorne Marlow, the VFW's director of Public Affairs. "That's just not so."

Regardless of sentiments like those from Olson and Marlow, Vietnam veterans were pleased when Congress approved monies for the special program. "It's belated, but it's needed," said a former officer of the National Association of Concerned Veterans, a group composed mainly of younger veterans.

The program itself is housed in about ninety informal storefront locations around the country. They are staffed by three or four counselors, usually Vietnam veterans themselves, and it is hoped the setting, *purposefully advertised as being physically removed from any VA hospital or facility,* will lure otherwise skeptical veterans in for help. "These guys have been burned or turned off by the VA," says one counselor in the West. "Maybe we can get things straightened out for them if they don't connect us directly with the VA."

Very few, if any, VA markings or other identifying symbols are visible at the storefronts. The VA as the funding source is obscured and ties to the agency are played down. Thus, in an overdue attempt to help an era's veterans, the VA simultaneously announces for all to see the depths of its arrogance in its claims that it is offering, over the years, the best care available.

Basically, the workers at the neighborhood offices, which fifteen years ago were considered to be an innovative attempt to bring psychiatric assistance to consumers rather than have them wade through hospital waiting lines and bureaucracy, will serve as liaisons between the veterans and appropriate agencies—including the VA. They will also offer a setting for veterans just to come in and rap about their war-related experiences. And their civilian aftermath.

But as noble and as needed as these services most definitely are, they omit the basic ingredient that made them so successful almost two decades ago. Although most clients back then were not veterans, a smattering of Vietnam servicemen did come through the storefront doors operated by the Lincoln Hospital Mental Health Services in the South Bronx, one of the pioneers in the field.

And any success that program had must be chalked up to the mix of workers available to help. Not only were local neighborhood mental health workers employed—indeed, they were the rock and foundation of the program—but so were psychologists, psychiatrists, nurses, and others.

No one individual because of his or her position, training, or background prevailed. But what did prevail was a difference in perspective among the workers, enabling those seeking help to draw upon a variety of mutually appropriate understandings, backed by the necessary clinical support, as needed. It worked well. And it is something the VA's readjustment program lacks. If, say, a physician is called for, the veteran will, after all is said and done, still have to go to the VA hospital, whence he had fled in the first place.

Don Crawford, the bearded thirty-nine-year-old Vietnam veteran picked by Cleland to head the program, acknowledges the legitimacy of his peers' criticism of the VA, and their wariness of the new setup. "Their anger is accurate but counterproductive," he says. "It makes for righteous indignation. While it may be truthful, it's not the way to get people on your side to help you.

"The VA and the military were as confused as anybody about what Vietnam was about," adds the freckle-faced Ph.D. in counseling who spent eighteen months in combat with the navy. In retrospect, he says, the violence, drugs, and personal problems the program is meant to cope with are reactions to guerrilla warfare circumstances encountered in Southeast Asia.

"But raising hell is not the way to enlist support. The way to do it is to raise the public's consciousness about what happened in Vietnam."

"Why the fuck should the VA get shit on?" is the way the chief, Psychology Division, at the Washington, D.C., hospital succinctly puts it. "It didn't make the goddamned war."

True enough. But the war refuses to go away. It lashes out everywhere. It was an international obscenity, now come home to roost in the form of Max Cleland's and Don Crawford's readjust-ment program, whether they liked it, or were ready for it, or not.

As with other wars, the blood and sweat from this one are mostly gone now. Just the tears remain, and the fury. As Jim Hebron can testify.

If there was any question about Hebron's anger and disgust over the long-distance wire from New York, this thirty-two-year-old director of the Veterans Advisement Center at the College of Staten Island and a decorated marine combat veteran in Vietnam didn't let the doubt linger.

"I'm really pissed. I'm goddamned furious." His ire was di-rected at the readjustment program. "It's fucked already," he ex-ploded. "It just started [October 1, 1979] and already the fucking thing is down the tubes. It's the same malaise.

"Crawford doesn't know what he's doing. Those assholes. It's the only goddamn program for us, the Vietnam veteran. The only one! They gave us ten million dollars. That's one percent of one point two billion dollars. One percent. And it's going down the tubes."

When Hebron, a handsome man with graying brown hair, is excited, his words tend to bump into each other, creating a strange New England rhythm that sounds as if it is being wrestled to the ground by his native Queens cadences.

He explains, rapid-fire, that people at the Brooklyn VA, the focus of the region's outreach efforts, are "rehiring the sameold-peoplewhodidn'tgiveadamnbefore. It's the same old cronyism." His letter to Cleland on this topic also exudes his breathless inten-sity.

"The bush league tactics . . . serve as grist for the mill for Vietnam veterans' assertions that the VA is an insensitive, insular and self-serving institution," he writes. "A natural by-product of this is to further alienate, frustrate and anger an already abused veteran population."

Citing what he says is Crawford's "indifference," Hebron pleads, "Max, you've got to know that the veterans in New York are really angry about what's happening. They really feel that the only large scale national program for the Vietnam veteran that is worth a damn is going down for the third and perhaps final time."

He takes a breath, and apologizes for displaying his anger on the phone.

From a welfare family not unfamiliar with the vagaries of a large bureaucracy, Hebron in many ways symbolizes the commitment and integrity of the men and women who fought a war only to find, on their return, that they were no longer needed. Hanging outside Hebron's office-cubicle at the College of Staten Island, from where he is calling, is a red, white, and blue sign. On it is a quote from the French philosopher Albert Camus: "I should like to be able to love my country and still love justice."

Jim Hebron was a young marine recruit at Khe Sanh during the 1968 Tet offensive. He was an infantryman and scout sniper, not yet twenty years old, and he is thankful to have escaped alive. In his scrapbook he keeps a frayed March 18, 1968, issue of *Newsweek*. The cover story details the terror of his combat unit under siege during the Tet assault. Hebron points to the photos and counts off his buddies who didn't survive.

"The whole thing was a sense of betrayal," he says. "Not just the VA.

"I was walking through the Los Angeles airport at two in the morning," he remembers. "There were six of us, all in uniform. There were some hippie couples at the time. This was '68, flower children. This young girl asked me how many children did I kill? Holy shit! I had just come back and that's what I got. Did they give a shit at home? I didn't commit any atrocities. And I didn't know anybody who committed any atrocities."

The VA, he suggests, had the same attitude.

"I thought when I got out of the service, I'd get a free education, go to college for free. I'm a veteran. It's going to be great, man. They told me that when I enlisted at sixteen. I was really a young kid. I believed everything that they told me. It was just over four years later, when I got out—well, the reality's a lot different. A hundred and seventy-five dollars doesn't buy you crap."

Hebron, like millions of his Vietnam-era comrades, discovered that GI educational benefits were not as advertised. After World

War II, returning veterans were entitled to benefits for tuition, fees, and book expenses plus a monthly stipend of sixty dollars. This enabled the veteran to attend any approved institution of higher education regardless of tuition costs.

In contrast, the Vietnam-era veteran received only a monthly stipend that didn't even begin to approach covering the increased costs of education. As a result, after WW II, schools like Harvard and Notre Dame had veteran populations of 59 percent and 85 percent, respectively, compared with 2 percent after Vietnam.

The VA likes to boast that the "participation rate" for educational benefits among Vietnam-era veterans increased to 64.8 percent in 1978, compared with 50.5 percent for veterans trained under the WW II program. The VA even totes up the billions of dollars expended and finds "post–Korean conflict trainees" to have received almost twice that allotted the earlier veterans.

The VA, however, conveniently overlooks the fact that far fewer Vietnam vets have *completed* the education they set out to get and that fewer still never get beyond a semester or two at most. In fact, many vets, unable to find a job, apply for educational benefits just to keep body and soul together, without attending one class. And those who do go to school tend to enroll at junior and community colleges, where the tuition is less—and the education limited.

In short, the VA figures are misleading. And a whole new underclass of alienated, unemployed citizens, rejected once they are no longer needed, swells the ranks of the underfunded social welfare agencies.

Even those who do follow through, as Hebron did, have their patience tested. It took him two years, and three semesters of being forced to drop out of school for lack of funds, before he straightened out the payment schedule fouled up by the VA. "I finally got it resolved through a friend of mine at the VA," he says. "It took him twenty-five minutes to clear it up. That really pissed me off.

"I guess I'm a cynic at this point," Hebron continues, "but I didn't expect bad things from the VA at first because it was a civilian agency. But they shuffle your papers as callously as any four-star general. I have no respect for anybody who works at the VA."

He's not the only one. And many, like Jim Hebron, inevitably personalize their anger.

"Cleland is selling us down the river," insists Peter Theys, forty-eight, seventeen years on active duty and now the DAV service officer at Gadsden, Alabama.

"He's a triple amputee. We thought he'd fight for us. He really let us down. He's nothing but a yes man for the president. And I'd tell him that right to his face."

Ralph Casteel, more than three decades as a top assistant to a variety of VA chiefs and currently a staff member of the powerful House Committee on Veterans' Affairs, puts it much more colorfully.

"I have no use for Max Cleland. He's never raised one finger of his good hand against OMB or President Carter. He doesn't know what the hell's going on out there in the field. If Carter says 'Shit,' Cleland will break his good arm getting his belt unbuckled and [former Chief Medical Director] Crutcher would be in the amen corner."

Thorne H. Marlow, director of public affairs for the almost two-million-member Veterans of Foreign Wars, sums it up: "We don't even deal with Mr. Cleland anymore."

For the ordinary veteran, however, the VA and its officials cannot be dismissed so easily.

It is 1:30 on a July afternoon and the Hardee's Charbroiled Hamburger outlet overlooking Interstates 75–85 in Atlanta is filled with thirsty and hungry Georgia Tech customers. Ken Baker, a two-tour Vietnam army combat veteran, wheels onto the driveway and parks his small gas-saver in the store's parking lot.

Baker walks into the eating place, sees the long lines in front of the counter, turns, and walks out.

Driving over to the nearby Varsity, where he quickly gets two hot dogs and a soft drink to go, he sighs irritably and says, "I'm tired of waiting on lines. I waited on lines in the army and I waited on lines at the VA. I'm not going to wait on lines when I want to eat." Baker, an intense, quiet-spoken man with a soft, pleasant Georgia accent, has been waiting on lines of one kind or another for more than eleven years, dating back prior to his honorable discharge on June 3, 1968.

He says he has tinnitus, subjective ringing in the ears, resulting from his prolonged proximity to artillery—106-mm. recoilless rifles—during combat. A constant, relentless companion, the tinnitus is so painful that Baker, thirty-three, cannot sleep unless he drugs himself with unprescribed depressants.

The increasing psychological distress from the continuous excruciating pain is compounded by the VA's refusal to acknowledge that the tinnitus occurred while Baker was in the service—or even to acknowledge his psychological discomfort.

"They're saying to me, 'Prove it. Did you go see a doctor, did you see a psychiatrist back in 1968 or '69?' I was so goddamned happy to be where nobody was shooting at me and where there were pretty girls walking around with their titties bouncing, I could have cared less. Plus, I had things on my mind, schoolwork and other stuff I had to do.

"When I got out of the service, they give you a separation physical. You know, put the earphones on, the guy says, 'Push the button when you hear the sound.' Well, I put on the earphones and immediately pushed the button all the way down. The guy says, 'I'm sorry, you can't do that.' I said, 'Well, you said you wanted me to hear the sound. I heard a sound. I always hear sounds.' He sent me over to the army hospital for an additional hearing examination. The guy never made the sound with his machine."

The pressures of his situation came to a head in January 1979, "when I made a commitment to turn off my brain to try and stop the ringing." His friends, alarmed at his condition, suggested he go to the VA. He had long since quit his teaching job of six years and had already gone through a brief stint as a 7-11 store clerk. He stays away now from loud places—bars, clubs, crowds.

He didn't work at all for fourteen months in 1977 and 1978.

"Where am I supposed to have gotten the tinnitus, except Vietnam?"

So in December 1978, Baker went to the VA for help. "I knew I was having a problem. I just needed to talk to a shrink. And being unemployed, I couldn't afford to go to a private shrink. So I thought I'd go to the VA."

He got initiated quickly. "You can't do anything at the VA without having to wait."

Baker finally got to see a young clerk who asked what the problem was. He told her he needed to see a psychiatrist.

"She says, 'What about?' I said if I knew I wouldn't need to see a psychiatrist.

"She said, 'Well, you can explain it to me.'

"I said, 'I don't understand it myself and I doubt seriously if the psychiatrist will understand it.'

"'Well, our procedures . . .'

"I said, 'Lady, I'm not going to stand up, jump across this table and bash you in the face just to prove I'm crazy.' And I got up and walked out.

"But I had to convince some technician that I was mentally ill before I could even see the shrink."

Without the sought-after help, his concerns persisted.

"There are two things that've really got me bothered. One is that in moments of extreme intensity I keep having the thought that I really ought to take one of my rifles off the wall and just kill a bunch of folks. That way they'll know I'm crazy, and they'll deal with me. The other thing is when I'm very depressed, I really wonder if it's worth it. I have no future, I'm not enjoying the present. . . . I have a basic philosophy that I came too close to dying, but it bothers me that I occasionally sit there and think to myself that there's no reason to go on."

Since February 1979, Baker has been employed as a veteran counselor for the Veterans Outreach Project of Economic Opportunity Atlanta, Inc. He is also in the process of a second appeal of the VA's refusal to acknowledge, and provide compensation for, the service-connected origin of the tinnitus.

Both endeavors are a strain on his own energies.

"If the VA decides, well, sorry, we can't deal with this, then just to feed myself, I have got to continue working in an environment where at least once a week or once every two weeks, I got to sit down and use the strength that I'm trying to use to hold my shit together to help some fella that's crazier than I am that's having problems with the VA worse than I ever dreamed of.

"Now, if you're a triple amputee like Max Cleland, the VA bends over backwards. You got any visible problems, they take care of you. I'd been better off if I had been shot—physical evidence, red badge of courage, something like that.

"Apparently, if I wind up getting screwed because of this, I'm gonna get screwed because I don't lose my cool. You know, when I was in the paratroopers and they told me I'm gonna have to run that five miles, whether you want to or not, you just endure, you do it.

"That's part of what got developed in my personality—I just endure. Because I've got problems and someone else is stupid, that's no reason why I should ruin his life. But because I haven't done that, because I haven't gone out of my way to prove to the rest of the world that I'm crazy, I may end up getting the shaft."

In May 1979, Max Cleland declared a time of national honoring of the men and women who fought the country's most recent war. Seizing the opportunity, Baker, who in 1977 had garnered 8,000 votes in a bid for a seat on the Atlanta school board, tried getting some help and respect.

He wound up in a line again.

"During Vietnam Veterans Week," he says, "the VA hospital here in town had an open house. Let the public see the VA at work, honor the vets, that sort of thing. So as part of my job I showed up out there.

"As I was starting to walk in, I was asked, 'Are you a veteran?' I said, 'As a matter of fact, I am.' 'Well, veterans have to sign in at the table.' There was a line at the table.

"So, I'm on line ten minutes to sign in to an open house. Only the VA can make veterans stand in line for an open house. I couldn't believe it. I told several people, and they didn't seem to see the irony of it."

Still, Baker was treated better than many other veterans at the hospital, a light-blue and white brick structure perched on a slight grassy knoll overlooking Clairmont Road in Decatur, a clean-cut suburb away from the confusion and congestion—and clientele—of downtown Atlanta.

Several feet in from the large sliding glass doors leading into the lobby, a woman at the information desk is busily scanning an advertising flyer of some sort. I tell her I would like to see the director. Incredibly, without missing a beat, she says she is "not allowed" to let anyone in to see the director but that "our medical director" is available.

"He's our PR person," she chirps.

In the medical director's office, the people bustling about cannot understand why I was brought there. Finally, someone suggest that I see "Mr. Grim—he handles our public relations."

The name fits, and if he handles their PR with the same aplomb with which he greeted an inquiring journalist, it's no wonder there are veterans running around thinking of blowing the place to smithereens.

Grim, it turns out, is the assistant director and a very busy man. He has thinning black hair, combed tightly against his white scalp. He wears his VA ID badge attached to the left lapel of his green suit jacket. He has been with the VA since 1945.

I explain who I am, why I'm there, and that I would understand if he didn't have time to see me since I just walked in without an appointment. He assures me that he does have a few minutes, but as I start to ask him questions, it becomes clear that he's realized he has made a mistake, after all.

I want to know about the hospital's policy toward Vietnam veterans.

"Of course we treat all veterans," he says. "We place special emphasis on the Vietnam veteran, of course." Then he says, "I don't think I have much to say. I don't really think I have the time to sit here and talk with you. Why don't you go to Washington? Talk to them there."

"I already did."

"Well, I'm busy. The hospital director is leaving for Washington tomorrow and I've got things to do."

"Can I call you to set up an appointment to see you?"

Panic. And anger. The temperature of the cool air-conditioned room goes up a few degrees.

"I don't think I have anything to say that you couldn't find out in Washington," he concludes grimly.

Downstairs in the pharmacy, which is not air-conditioned, about forty people are waiting in olive-green cushioned chairs. They look up frequently at the board above the pharmacy window to see if their number has lit up. Over the window, to the left of the call display, a sign reads: "Service-connected veterans are given priority service."

Hanging from the wall to the right of the number-board is a fourteen-inch color television. Most people look at the number-board, not the TV.

The pharmacy in a VA hospital is a good place to get a rough feel for the operation of the facility. If there are few people waiting, the director tends to run an efficient, perhaps even relatively sensitive, enterprise within the allotted resources. In addition, people sitting around with nothing to do talk about their experiences at the hospital. If you listen, you can learn a lot.

A young, moustachioed Vietnam veteran who limps is the center of some attention in the rear of the waiting area. He is wearing a T-shirt: "Peaches—records and tapes." He is saying, "It's much better here now. Used to be you just set, but now they got the TV, so you don't mind waiting so much."

Another man, elderly and dressed in a neat business suit, has been sitting there all day. From his seat in the outpatient clinic, he can watch the activities in the Admissions and Evaluation section. Mainly, he sees patients being examined against regulations in the hallway, which is congested with large beds with wheels.

"I'm not coming here anymore," he says to a buddy who has spotted him. "I work. I can't wait all day. I'm gonna go to another hospital—let them come and get me."

If plans go according to schedule, a new ambulatory care wing should be in place in April 1982. Clearly, Max Cleland has not played favorites with VA facilities in his, and President Carter's, native state.

And, just as clearly, Ken Baker knows what he is getting into. He is hoping, though, that despite the odds, he may be able to hook up with someone like Robert K. Snyder, Assistant Veterans Service Officer at the Atlanta VA Regional Office (VARO), which is more centrally located than the hospital. Snyder, a former army captain, feels the Atlanta VARO offers better service because it's not as big as some of those situated in larger metropolitan areas.

But he has a problem when he has to offer the veteran what he describes as "all window dressing and not any substance."

He blames Cleland for not always following through coherently.

John Butler, the regional office's Veterans Benefits counselor responsible for prison and elderly outreach, and, like Snyder, committed and overworked, understands that "there is a social, psychological difference in the way the Vietnam veteran and the World War II veteran are looking at their military service."

These attitudes, he knows, can determine how a veteran relates to the VA. Ken Baker, for example.

"If the VA comes back negative," says Baker, finishing his second hot dog, "I don't know what I'll do. I can't keep working, and you can't feed yourself if you can't work.

"I keep telling myself, and I hope it never happens, but if I have to go out, I'm gonna go out in style. The problem with that is, you know, how do you shoot the VA?

"I hold no animosity toward the apathetic bureaucrats and clerks with their blinders on. All they see is what's on their desk. They don't look at you. You go out and shoot twenty or thirty of those, it won't do you any good.

"That's the problem. You just can't get at it. My case doesn't seem to fit into what their rules say. Therefore, the hell with it. If I don't fit into your procedures, don't tell me to go away. Change your goddamn procedures.

"The only thing that's saving the VA's ass right now is that Vietnam veterans, especially combat veterans, are basically loners.

"If all the combat veterans ever got together and said, 'Look, I don't give a shit what the world says, we're going to change the VA,' they would have to activate the army, and then it would be a long drawn-out procedure with the army suffering heavy casualties because ain't nobody in the army got half the experience we got. It would be awful."

Actually, the question is not one of shooting the VA. The more salient question is, How do you sue the VA?

The answer: You can't.

Knowing that, the explosive frustration directed toward the VA makes a whole lot more sense. As incredible as it may be, the fact is that the United States Veterans Administration is the only federal agency whose decisions are not subject to court review!

It has, in the process, become a law unto itself, a legally insulated old fogey where the lives of veterans, and their families, are at the tender mercies of an "outlaw" organization.

Under existing statutes, a local VA board reviews a veteran's case to determine eligibility for disability compensation, pension, and other benefits. If the local board rules against the veteran, he or she is permitted to appeal to the Washington, D.C.–based VA Board of Veterans Appeals. In effect the "Supreme Court" of the VA, the BVA is made up of some fifty members appointed by the president. Generally, the BVA hears veterans' appeals in panels of three members, usually consisting of a lawyer, a physician, and another with related expertise. Virtually all members have held prior positions in the VA hierarchy.

Periodically, the board holds hearings in various parts of the country, so that a veteran unable to make the trip to Washington can wait until the traveling board meets at a VA facility nearby. The veteran can also opt to have the appeal heard by three regional office employees, who will then send the hearing transcript to Washington for a decision.

It is an immense workload. Each member is often responsible for deciding upward of fifteen hundred appeals a year. Only one in eight appeals is won, even though the hearings are supposedly nonadversary and "reasonable doubt" must be resolved in favor of the veteran.

And the veteran is prevented by law from going to court after he has exhausted the VA's appeal process.

In addition, although a veteran may bring along an attorney or representative to the appeal hearings, the attorney is not permitted to charge the veteran, under penalty of criminal law, *more than ten dollars*—and that only if the veteran wins the claim! Equally amazing is the fact that all the veterans' service organizations, along with the VA, have hysterically supported, strongly, this abrogation of a citizen's rights.

A closer look, however, reveals why the iron triangle—the VA, the service groups, and the Congress—has vigorously stuck to the startling notion that veterans, adults and free men all—somehow shorn of their constitutional prerogatives—must have government protection to save them from becoming the helpless prey of shyster lawyers.

If veterans can't get adequate legal representation (and for ten bucks, God knows, they can't), then to whom do they turn?

The VFW and American Legion, that's who. Housed in the VA facilities themselves, these organizations, touted as the friends of the veteran, accompany veterans to the hearings free of charge. When dues-paying time next rolls around, the grateful vet forks over a few dollars to the group that has helped him get, or try to get, his compensation.

Voilà, instant membership increase.

And, since the rate of dismissed or rejected appeals is so high, the VA and Congress figure, why take chances with letting some pushy, money-grubbing lawyer get in on the act?

It was a cozy arrangement—until 1979.

Under Max Cleland's leadership, the VA has urged Congress to change the law. In fact, Cleland's commitment was so strenuous that he brought in a Colorado attorney for the express purpose of guiding some meaningful modifications of the statute through the House and Senate. Dean Phillips, active over the past few years in this effort, and the VA finally witnessed some success when in September 1979 the Senate passed S-330, the VA's adjudication Procedure and Judicial Review Act. The House has yet to act on it, and supporters of the bill are pessimistic. Additionally, the American Legion, the nation's largest and most powerful veterans' group, is still dead set against the legislation.

The bill, if passed as voted on in the Senate, would provide for judicial review of the administrative decisions of the VA, and allow the payment of reasonable attorneys' fees. For the first time in more than half a century, the VA, almost three-quarters of whose budget is spent on those nonjudicially reviewable benefits claims (around $15 billion), has taken a giant step toward joining the rest of America's democratic institutions.

"The fundamental issue . . . is one of simple justice," asserts former Massachusetts Congress member Robert Drinan, the sponsor of legislation in the House. "To deny a citizen access to an attorney, to isolate an agency from the scrutiny of the courts, runs counter to the most basic precepts of our constitutional form of government.

"In my view, this legislation is long overdue."

In August 1979, Ken Baker wrote to me.

Yesterday I got the letter from the VA. They turned down my appeal.

Again I am dismayed that the VA has chosen to serve itself rather than a veteran. They have concentrated their logic on the tinnitus and have apparently ignored the psychological aspects of my case. It seems they have taken advantage of my mistake in first filing my claim.

In my ignorance, I claimed for ringing in the ears (which is, I believe, still at the root of my problems), rather than seeking proper advice. When, during the hearing, the psychological aspects were added, the VA apparently chose not to acknowledge it. Their reasons for denial do not even mention problems other than tinnitus. The VA made no effort to help me; they simply chose the surest way to deny my claim.

To appeal further? I am not certain. . . . They just do not see what they do not wish to see. I have no faith in the VA to miraculously become benign between now and the next time they go into seclusion to exercise their exotic logic.

. . . I now know that I need help if I am to survive. I am saddened that the VA cannot be the source of that help. I am saddened that the VA has made no offer of medical help. But I shall try to do something; I have no choice.

Keep the faith,
Ken

> I don't think they could put him in a mental hospital. On the other hand, if he were already in, I don't believe they'd let him out.
> —*Charles van Kriedt*

8
PILL PUSHING AND DOPE DEALING

Scrawled in blue ink on the outside cover of Robert Shadron's Mountain Bell telephone book is the phone number of the White House in Washington, D.C. Although he has called Jimmy Carter's residence on several occasions, he has yet to speak with the president. But Shadron, a thirty-eight-year-old Marine Corps veteran now living in Phoenix, has communicated in writing with the Oval Office—as well as with virtually every member of the Senate and House, the FBI, the Justice Department, and a variety of Veterans Administration officials.

"I reported to your hospital on November 25, 1974, for purposes of examination and observation," he wrote on December 9, to one of those officials, the director of the Houston VA Medical Center. Three days earlier, Shadron, unemployed, had escaped from the psychiatric section of the facility, which he had entered voluntarily less than two weeks before.

"Upon my arrival at the hospital," the handwritten letter continues, "my clothes were taken, along with all my belongings, and I was taken to Ward 512 and locked up for ten days and nights. I was given injections which knocked me out, and medication, all against my will.

"When I asked to talk with a doctor concerning my injections, I was attacked by three men, one of which strangled me from behind and forced me to the floor where they injected me against my will. I feel that I am very lucky to have escaped from the hospital and be alive. . . ."

Shadron, whose father is a disabled World War II veteran, was sent, at his own request, to Houston for what was supposed to be a period of observation and examination for a *physical* condition, Dercum's disease. Instead, Shadron asserts, he was summarily locked in the psychiatric ward and massively dosed with Thorazine, a powerful tranquilizer used for highly agitated patients.

With the administration of the drug, Shadron, chosen as a marine recruit to lead his battalion in the boot camp graduation parade, was put on treatment status despite being voluntarily admitted to the facility for nontreatment purposes related to his disability claim.

He was, at that point, committed.

But for a patient to be committed to a psychiatric facility, legal steps, including a court hearing within twenty-four hours, must be taken. However, a signed, handwritten note from an attorney connected with a Washington, D.C., law firm, which did some preliminary investigation at Shadron's request, states, "I called Houston Probate Court and was told that there is no record of any commitment proceeding in that court between November 25, 1974, and December 16, 1975."

Those dates encompass Shadron's stay at the hospital.

In addition, Texas law also requires next of kin or a legal representative to be informed by registered mail when involuntary confinement occurs. Shadron says his family was never contacted by the hospital. Shadron, with two young children and a wife employed as a nurse by the VA, adds that during most of the time in Houston, one of the VA's largest hospitals, he slept on the

floor of a locked room, in various states of medicated consciousness.

He says, too, that another patient was injected with Thorazine
while he lay unconscious.

Although he had earlier experienced a serious negative reaction to drugs similar in chemical makeup to Thorazine—information documented in his VA file—Shadron continued to receive
against his will as much as 200 milligrams four times a day, even
though he told them of his prior allergic reaction.

The clinical psychologist who tested him at Houston noted in
his report that "[Shadron] had been withdrawn from Librium
[another tranquilizer] and placed on Thorazine prior to testing
and at one point he became so lethargic that the examination
had to be interrupted for a few days until he became more
alert." The psychologist added that the test results showed "definite signs of serious mental and emotional disturbance . . . signs
of paranoid thinking and preoccupation with violence and
gloom (suggesting) a paranoid psychotic disorder with depressive features."

Two days after the testing, Shadron escaped from what he
calls "illegal imprisonment" and the unsubstantiated charges in
his confidential VA records that he is "considered to be dangerous." Typical of Shadron's VA-related problems, a medical doctor
has inserted in parentheses, "This is not explained," after the
"dangerous" allegation.

In addition, Shadron contends he was never diagnosed paranoid prior to Houston, nor has he been so labeled since, despite
repeated examinations by psychiatrists and psychologists, including an exam at the Audie Murphy VA Medical Center in San
Antonio. Neither has he been dangerous or violent.

But he has been repeatedly turned down for his service-connected disability claim.

His efforts to expose what he insists to be civil and criminal
law violations at the Houston VA have likewise been shunted
aside or specifically denied. "It's easy when they call you schizophrenic," he says. VA officials deny his allegations, and then-FBI
director Clarence Kelley never responded to Shadron's plea to

"properly seek out those who are injuring our disabled veterans on Ward 512."

He calls it a cover-up.

"Whatever is convenient for them, that's what they do," he charges.

In May 1977, Shadron wrote to President Carter.

"The indiscriminate drugging in doses many times the maximum therapeutic dosage caused many veterans to suffer with overt signs of tranquilizing drug poisonings such as cogwheel rigidity, drooling, and shuffling gait," he told the president. "Many others were subjected to intense [summer] heat [in excess of 100 degrees Fahrenheit] in violation of the proper use of the drugs being administered."

He received no response.

"You know," Shadron says with bitterness and disgust, "I didn't have much sympathy with blacks, and the problems they said they had. If you riot, you deserved to be shot, I used to think. But I understand their position now. Frustration can be enormous when you can't get anyone to listen to common sense.

"Maybe soon only just people will be in prison. The average guy doesn't want to perpetuate this system. But the way things are, he might be just as well off on welfare than in the VA."

The Lyons VA Medical Center is an 1,100-bed psychiatric facility in bucolic Somerset County, New Jersey, not far from the state capital at Trenton. The hospital, which provides medical and nursing home care for its patients, is one of the system's older service components. It is divided into two clusters of buildings, called Circles, joined by tunnels. One Circle is composed only of psychiatric and substance abuse units; the other contains administrative offices, admissions office, the canteen, and other services.

Because of the center's age, the VA has been called on to deny there are plans afoot to close the facility. In fact, the hospital's future seems assured, as Congress heard in testimony in early 1979, by the move to expand its mandate into a general medical and surgery operation.

Right now, however, the medical center's past is what concerns many veterans at Lyons.

George Falter is one of them.

Falter, a fifty-five-year-old army vet with three years of infantry action in the Mediterranean and European theaters, was admitted to a closed ward in March 1977. Since then, he says he has been prevented from visiting a fellow patient in another building; patients and visitors have not been allowed to visit him; his mail has been withheld and interfered with; his right to withdraw his own funds, held by the hospital in an account, has been limited; and he frequently has been subjected to—and has been asked to feed others—cold, unrecognizable, and inedible food.

Robert Mahler is another.

Mahler, sixty-one, served four years while carrying out fifty-five bombing missions as a pilot in the "Flying Tiger" unit in the South China combat zone during World War II. Since 1978, Mahler, the holder of two Distinguished Flying Crosses, has been a patient at the Lyons nursing home.

From the time of his admission, he says, he has never been informed of his rights as a patient; his attorneys and other visitors have been subjected to questioning about the nature of their visits; and he has been interrogated, intimidated, and harassed by ward staff concerning those visits.

In addition, he claims his own personal possessions have been searched, repeatedly and without permission, by ward personnel; and, with the knowledge and acquiescence of the hospital staff, patients have been allowed to defecate and urinate in his room during a one-year period.

Frank Hubert (not his real name), a twenty-one-year-old navy veteran, was transferred to Lyons on October 3, 1978, from Trenton Psychiatric Hospital. The VA has found him to be disabled with a service-connected emotional disorder. After spending six months on both open and closed wards, Hubert was discharged on April 4, 1979. Three months later, in July, he was arrested by local police, brought to Ward 55C, and held there involuntarily.

Medical staff then forcibly injected him with powerful psychotropic medications, probably Thorazine, stripped him of his clothing and all his possessions, and restrained and treated him in a humiliating manner. At least once he was placed in leather cuffs because he demanded the right to call his attorney.

Hubert was released from the hospital after nine hours. No charges were preferred by the police.

On August 1, 1979, Falter, Mahler, Hubert, and three others filed a class-action lawsuit in U.S. District Court in New Jersey. They asked relief, for themselves and those in similar conditions, from the various deprivations and injuries they say they have experienced—including the right to attend religious services, the right to possess stamps and envelopes, and the right not to be physically threatened.

The suit, perhaps the first of its kind, was prepared by the New Jersey Public Advocate's office. It seeks a federal order mandating the VA to restore the constitutional rights of VA patients and ensure them adequate, responsible, and judicially enforced health care. The list of abuses, fourteen causes of action in all, includes those pertaining to cruel and unusual punishment, the right to privacy, and the free exercise of religion.

Patients, the suit alleges, "who complain to staff about these denials are frequently punished with isolation, restraints, or medication. Both ingoing and outgoing mail is deliberately delayed, destroyed or opened when deemed appropriate by ward staff, without the prior consent of the patient involved."

"They seem to have violated every civil right in the book," says William F. Culleton, Jr., the assistant deputy public advocate involved in the proceedings.

Robert Hegler, who doesn't know Culleton, kept a diary of his eight-month experience as an attendant at Lyons. He writes, "A veteran of this war was tied to a chair with a sheet. One of the attendants told him to shut up. When the patient refused, the attendant threw several punches into him. Five other attendants, including a head attendant, looked on without comment.

"The same night . . . I saw another attendant hit a young, non-resistive patient in the back . . . and hit him on two different occasions while he was in bed. Two weeks later, I was ordered by the head attendant to turn cold water on a patient held forcibly under a shower."

Hegler's detailed diary goes on to recount no less than fifty such instances of abuse. He tells of patients who were "wrung out"—choked with a towel—and of at least one patient who was held down by an attendant while being kicked in the head by another, eventually requiring stitches to mend the wound.

A seriously ill man beaten up by attendants while in bed, Hegler writes, died the following day. And Hegler tells the story of a nurse who angrily tossed medicine into a patient's face because he refused to finish taking it.

These abuses are not listed in Bill Culleton's lawsuit.

Robert Hegler's diary, as contemporary as it seems, was written in 1945.

About two months after Hegler's revelations, which were originally reported in the New York *Journal-American,* the VA issued a statement conceding the presence of abuses and promising a cleanup. "The investigation," the VA eventually announced, "reveals some substantiation of the charges made by Robert Hegler. The abuses were to a considerable degree due to . . . untrained and inefficient attendant help and inadequate coverage of the wards.

"Appropriate steps are being taken," the statement promised, "to remedy the situation as to the attendant group, as well as certain changes in the professional and sub-professional groups."

The New Jersey patients are still waiting, thirty-five years later. Aside from the transfer of the physician in charge to another building at Lyons ("But he's no longer on the acute wards," cooed chief of staff Col. L. V. Lopez), no one was punished for the conditions at the hospital.

Which brings us to the present.

Like his esteemed predecessor of three and a half decades ago, former President Carter's VA administrator Cleland promised, too, to make things better for the veterans at Lyons. (If nothing else, the VA is consistent in its promises.)

On July 14, 1978, Arthur Penn, New Jersey's deputy commissioner in the Department of the Public Advocate, wrote to Cleland. Penn's letter was in response to an earlier missive from Cleland in which the VA boss acknowledged he saw "merit" in the state's position that VA regulations concerning patient care be upgraded to the more progressive and humane levels of New Jersey's statutes.

Cleland also had written that a Patients' Bill of Rights, hard to come by at Lyons (and elsewhere), was at that time being worked on. "In the interim," wrote Cleland, "rest assured that I, as well as my General Counsel and Chief Medical Director, will see that the civil rights of our patients will continue to be protected."

Penn didn't rest assured. In his response to Cleland, Penn offered the help of his office in writing the new regulations. As the suit pointed out, without posted rights, patients had very little basis on which to determine the fairness and applicability of the hospital regulations and their enforcement. (The Albuquerque VA, for example, went for months without a patient handbook, thereby making it difficult to know what the hospital's rules were, and the administration's parameters for enforcement.)

Penn also outlined the patients' complaints and asked Cleland to appoint a specific person at both the Lyons and East Orange VA facilities with whom problems could be discussed.

Penn never heard from Cleland again.

On September 5, Penn tried once more. He wrote to the VA director, reminding him of the situation at Lyons. He added that "it is clear that further delay [in dealing with patients' complaints of civil rights violations] would be unreasonable." Promises notwithstanding, Cleland followed the well-worn path of his 1940s counterpart. So far, things have not, in fact, improved at Lyons; the VA responded to the suit, denying everything.

"Things in the VA don't change much over the years, do they?" asks a government official familiar with the history of the Lyons VA.

Nor do they change much from state to state.

For Mac McNairy, a sixty-nine-year-old widower placed and detained involuntarily for four months in 1977 at the Brentwood VA psychiatric hospital in Los Angeles, there was no question of his rights being violated. Without his eyeglasses, he couldn't have read them even if they were put directly in front of him (which they weren't).

Sarah Jongepier, of the Southern California American Civil Liberties Union medical complaint center, visited McNairy after hearing of his plight through a local TV program.

She went to the ward with her husband, Neil, also on the ACLU staff. "There was a nurse on duty, like a guard, screening people coming in and going out," Sarah Jongepier recalls. "We asked if we could see Mr. McNairy, and we gave her our identification. She said absolutely not.

"We said, 'We have the permission of the patient.' She said, 'That doesn't make any difference.' We asked her to bring him to the door and let him tell us in her presence whether he wants to see us or not. She said no, she wouldn't call the patient.

"At that point, we saw a patients' bill of rights posted on the bulletin board across the hall, so we walked over and said, 'Well, how do you explain that, the fact the patient is allowed to have visitors at the patient's discretion?' And she just couldn't explain it."

The Jongepiers asked to speak with someone else. The nurse directed them to the medical officer of the day. He informed them that the VA's patients cannot be visited by the media or a legal organization without the hospital's permission.

"We asked to see the patients' bill of rights," Sarah Jongepier says. "He looked through all his books and said, 'The bill of rights must be around here someplace.' But he couldn't quite determine where it was and besides, those were the hospital's rules."

Pushed, the medical officer finally agreed to have McNairy examined by a staff doctor "to see if he is capable of having visitors." The Jongepiers went along, reluctantly. But it turned out the doctor chosen to do the examination—the psychiatric emergency admitting physician—somehow never did find the time to look at McNairy. "So we left."

Sarah Jongepier says that because he was a probate conservatee (basically a ward of the state), "I knew that Mr. McNairy should not be in a mental ward against his will. And Mr. McNairy obviously was on a locked mental ward against his will."

She explains that McNairy was placed in Brentwood through the neglect of the Los Angeles County public guardian's office, and that the VA compounded the error when it accepted him without going through the legal process necessary to commit an involuntary patient. As a result, the ACLU initiated a class-action suit on behalf of McNairy "and all others similarly situated" against LA County.

But the VA was intractable.

"Mr. McNairy had no psychiatric history, so I wondered why he was being kept there," Sarah Jongepier continues. "Since I also knew he was a probate conservatee, I knew he was wrongfully placed and he wanted out and they wouldn't let him out. So there was no doubt about it that under these circumstances, he needed an attorney."

Jongepier got him an attorney.

"We asked to have a private place to meet with him on the ward, and the staff very grudgingly told us we could meet in the library. But at least we finally convinced them he could see visitors if he wished. The first thing we did was have him sign a statement allowing the ACLU to see his records. He didn't have his glasses, so we wrote the statement in big letters, and he signed it after reading it back to us.

"We hadn't been there more than five minutes when a social worker dropped in. She wanted to change the venetian blinds. It wasn't more than another five minutes later when another social worker came in and sat down. We asked her to leave. But we just had a terrific time getting everybody out of the room so we could talk with him privately.

"So we had a very brief and kind of a harassed sort of situation, but we did meet with him."

Jongepier points out that, on TV, the hospital said he could leave whenever he wanted. "I knew he couldn't because of the travel distance involved and because he was so heavily drugged. He had no realistic way of getting home. He had no pocket money, no bus money, but they kept saying he could leave at any time he wants."

Finally in court, the judge immediately ordered McNairy

placed on a medical ward and his drugs reevaluated. "We found out he was on seven different prescription drugs," says Jongepier. "The court ordered those reduced and that his home be prepared for his return. He was in the VA for three months before it came to light on public TV. I wonder how many more like him the VA has on its psychiatric wards?"

It is virtually axiomatic that a nation's capacity for compassion is reflected in its attitudes toward the helpless in its midst: the poor, the maimed, the physically ill, the young, the emotionally handicapped. Add the psychiatrically disabled veteran to that list and you have a quick study of the powerless in this country.

In many respects, we do not know what to do with our "mental" patients. One week we offer them chemicals, the next it's behavior modification. And the week after that, group therapy. But the numbers of patients do not decrease significantly. And after wartime, they increase. The widespread use of drugs has masked the fact that, while there may be fewer patients occupying psychiatric beds than ever before, their emotional disturbance, now possibly blunted, is nonetheless still present.

We have traded a bed for a pill, and only the patient is the wiser. And the drug companies richer.

The VA brags of the innovations it has contributed to the care of psychiatric patients. True, the VA has almost single-handedly created the market for clinical and counseling psychologists by its early acceptance of the discipline in the 1940s. Right now, it is still the largest single employer of psychologists, though, much to the annoyance of many of them, it maintains their status at a Civil Service level while their M.D. brethren are exempt from the same kind of bureaucratic rigmarole.

The VA, too, points to its pioneering role in the use of psychotropic medications that have reduced the length of stay in psychiatric wards. Although the example at Brentwood might suggest VA policy is geared toward *increasing* the stay of patients, even nonpsychiatric ones, it is true that time spent in those wards has dropped dramatically.

In ten years, 1968–78, the VA has reduced the number of psychiatric patients from an average daily census of 47,883 to 22,836—a drop of more than 50 percent. During that same period, the average monthly turnover quadrupled—from 15.4 percent to 60.6 percent—and the number of patients treated jumped from 146,732 to 188,808 annually. For the period 1971–76, total discharges of patients with mental disorders went from 262,335 to 343,027.

The VA controls about 10 percent of all the psychiatric beds in the United States. In 1965, 59,000 (about 49 percent) of the VA's 120,000 beds were designated as psychiatric. In 1975, 29,827 (32 percent) of a total 94,477 operating VA beds were listed as psychiatric. Currently, 126 VA medical centers have psychiatric bed sections, including twenty-seven hospitals that predominantly treat a psychiatrically disturbed population.

Not surprisingly, most acute VA psychiatric care is available in urban areas (where medical school affiliations are present); most chronic psychiatric care beds are in rural areas (where affiliations are not present). Yet, regardless of where the veteran is located, the 1978 VA Patient Satisfaction Survey reveals that in every category monitored, including physician and nursing care, psychiatric patients clearly are less satisfied with their care throughout the system than are their medical and surgical counterparts. Especially pertinent is the emotional support category, which was rated favorable by slightly more than 50 percent of the medical and surgical patients as against approximately 40 percent of the psychiatric patients.

The figures would undoubtedly have been worse if the VA hadn't several years earlier followed through on its closure of surgical services in most of its psychiatric facilities and dramatically reduced the amount of surgery in others. The situation in those hospitals was so bad that the 1977 National Academy of Sciences study commissioned by the VA found that "even though the psychiatric hospitals perform less complicated procedures, the crude mortality rate for operations done in psychiatric hospitals in fiscal year 1975 was more than twice as high as the rate in general hospitals. . . . The rate is so much higher than in general hospitals that it must be cause for concern."

NAS recommended the removal of surgical services from those hospitals, a move the VA had already undertaken.

It is surprising, in fact, that the dissatisfaction rate of the VA's psychiatric population is not significantly higher, considering the evidence. Much of the VA's experimental research is done on psychiatric patients, a helpless and powerless group of individuals if there ever was one.

- In the 1950s, psychiatric patients at the Bronx VA were subjects in CIA-sponsored experiments involving the drug LSD.
- Ten years later, in the late 1960s, LSD experiments using schizophrenic alcoholics were run at the Sheridan VA in Wyoming.
- Psychosurgery, the technique of slicing away emotional centers of the brain which has been enthusiastically supported by the VA over the years, was being conducted into the late 1970s at places like Durham, Long Beach, Syracuse, and Minneapolis. Started in 1943 as an experimental procedure, it is still used by the VA, even though its benefits are questionable.
- The testing of new drugs is an ongoing practice, and VA psychiatric wards are major experimental settings for an array of exotic tranquilizers and so-called antipsychotic medications. In 1975, the GAO identified at least thirteen VA psychiatric sections where Thioridazine, a "zombie medicine" that can cause eye damage, was being overprescribed.
- Electroshock treatment, an extreme method of therapy for psychiatric patients, especially severely depressed ones, has been administered at Chicago's Downey VA hospital, without the consent of at least one of the patients involved.

"The majority of research, whether it be psychosurgery or experimentation with new drugs, is done on precisely those individuals who have the least to say about their destiny," Dr. Bernard Diamond, of the University of California Law School, testified in 1974 before Senator Edward Kennedy's committee hearings on human experimentation. "[They] tend to be dependent individuals . . . in no position to protest or complain."

Inadvertently supporting the charge leveled by Diamond and others in an attempt to rationalize the VA's position, Dr. Lawrence Hobson, a deputy for Research and Development at the VA, insists that veterans are "not dependent, except for some of the psychiatric patients. . . . They're free to leave whenever they want."

Data gathered by Hobson's own department do not fit in with that perspective. Approximately 70 percent of VA patients have no health insurance that adequately provides for medical treatment. Furthermore, psychiatric patients are even less likely to have access to third-party payments for health care. Therefore, it is clear that most—the vast majority, in fact—VA patients have no alternatives to VA medical treatment. Contrary to Hobson's uninformed analysis, they cannot "leave whenever they want" for the simple and obvious reason that they have nowhere else to go. Patients who feel pressured by medical and financial problems are less likely to object to entreaties to participate in medical experiments, particularly when those making the request have the power and authority to alter their treatment status.

"You always have to keep an eye out for the occasional individual who is a little too gung-ho about a particular research project and forgets that they're treating people," admits Dr. Joan Woods, staff psychiatrist at the Murfreesboro psychiatric VA hospital in Tennessee. "But the VA has safeguards," she quickly adds. "You can't just walk in today and decide you're going to do drug research and start doing it. I suspect right now we're probably erring on the side of not doing research that ought to be done. I think when I was in medical school, the patients were not sufficiently protected. I suspect right now they're overprotected."

"We encourage basic medical research of high quality in the VA," says Dr. Bette Uzman, chief of Medical Research for the entire VA. "We're constantly monitoring, but people aren't perfect. Site visits are important in this respect. They've been very effective."

The VA, of course, likes to offer statistics supportive of this attitude.

The 1978 VA annual report, for example, boasts of a study that measured the quality of care provided for long-term patients in twenty VA medical centers with large numbers of psychiatric beds. Drawing data from 3,500 patients on 240 wards, the results "reflect [the fact] that most patients are satisfied with the care they are receiving and have confidence in the staff." The report ignores the dependent status of these veterans, which makes the reliability of these results suspect. Further, the dubiousness of these numbers becomes apparent when it is noted that VA officials are quick to accept and promote the validity of these favorable responses while in the same breath warning that complaints and allegations must be viewed with skepticism—when they come from these same psychiatric patients.

It's hard to have it both ways, but the VA tries.

Informed that patients at the Albuquerque VA had been critical of his leadership, Joseph Birmingham, the hospital's director, responded. "From what I've seen, I'd be willing to bet you, dollars to doughnuts, that nine out of ten of the people who called in and who have had their cases followed up here have got mental health problems. And if that's the case, I can't comment on it."

Later, when several psychiatric patients made public their positive feelings about treatment there, the administration breathed a collective sigh of satisfaction. And Birmingham issued no caveats about the veracity of the testimony.

If name-calling doesn't produce the desired results, then invoking incompatible but damning diagnoses might.

In the case of one thirty-four-year-old Vietnam army private, the records reveal contradictory diagnoses within three weeks of each other. On one day his VA label is "hysterical neurosis, presumed." It is followed twenty-one days later by a psychologically incompatible "schizophrenia, chronic undifferentiated." Needless to add, the schizophrenia tag stuck.

Both diagnoses were wrong.

This particular veteran is earning a living and supporting himself very well, without help from the VA and without any signs of either hysterical neurosis (an outdated catchall phrase no longer used by most clinicians) or schizophrenia, chronic, undifferentiated, or otherwise.

The VA can also dig down into its bag of tricks and create before your very eyes a situation in which a psychiatric diagnosis is simply unavoidable, as it did with Tony Gonzales, the Vietnam vet who wound up in the psychiatric ward because the VA didn't get him a leg brace.

And if a veteran can't be dismissed for lack of psychiatric diagnosis, the VA may make one up.

In the latter part of 1977, C. Wayne Hawkins, director of the Dallas VA Medical Center, began receiving letters of complaint from William Crisler, the outspoken officer of a DAV chapter in Mesquite, Texas. The letters alleged unsanitary conditions and practices at the facility, suggested inadequacies in medical care, and asserted Crisler knew of drug thefts on the grounds. Crisler communicated some of these charges to Senator Cranston.

In a December 6, 1977, letter to Cranston, Hawkins strongly rejected the allegations, calling them "unfounded." Then, as if to emphasize his own credibility, Hawkins wrote at the end of the letter,

We are quite disturbed by Mr. Crisler's activities and the tone of his letters because they appear to indicate a serious psychiatric disturbance. He has *no history of mental illness* but a member of our psychiatry staff has reviewed his letters and believes he is a victim of "involutional psychosis" and may be dangerous. We plan to offer psychiatric help but are doubtful that Mr. Crisler will be receptive. [Italics added.]

Hawkins then offers this parting shot to the senator: "The above is supplied to you in your official capacity and should not be divulged to the veteran. We appreciate your interest in this case."

Crisler, who fought in more than one war, calls the letter "typical of the Gulag syndrome at the VA."

The rationale is quite simple: Psychiatric patients cannot be believed (at least not the complaining ones); if they cannot be believed, then charges of civil rights abuses and human rights violations can be ignored. The result: no rights at all, and, occasionally, no treatment, either.

Anyone who has ever worked in a psychiatric setting of any kind knows the ease—and, often, eagerness—with which a label is magnetically affixed, and the more extreme the label, the more difficult it is to erase. The person becomes a cipher, a category, summed up neatly if not arcanely by whatever the medical dictionary of the era happens to define as the prevailing symptoms. (For instance, *hysteria,* the Greek word for "uterus," was once identified by the presence of a wandering womb. The diagnosis was limited to women. Other segments of the population are given other labels.)

"A patient admitted and given a psychiatric diagnosis is stigmatized, simply because our society sees it that way," says Dr. Charles Stenger, associate director for psychology at the VA's central office. "That's not true of medical and surgical patients."

"While schizophrenia is considered a 'medical diagnosis' like pneumococcal pneumonia or appendicitis," writes Dr. Hugh Drummond, a psychiatrist, "it actually functions as a degradation ritual imposed upon those who have broken some rules of propriety. While the label is affixed with ease, it can never be removed. Innumerable times I have seen a thick medical record in which a medical student had once added schizophrenia to a list of possible diagnoses. Years later, an intern who has zipped through the chart will begin a note on the patient by writing, 'This is the fifth admission of a 48-year-old male schizophrenic.'

"Everyone concerned is thereby permitted to take the patient's complaints less seriously, which saves a lot of time and trouble. And if mental patients are anything, they are people about whom not much trouble is ever taken."

Not even the trouble to find out the accuracy or inaccuracy of the label.

Drummond, easily the most sensitive, sensible, and insightful doctor in print today (and, possibly, in any clinic as well), cites one study in which transcripts of normal speech were given to a group of psychiatrists. The speakers, unknown to the doctors, were simply identified as patients, and the psychiatrists were asked to diagnose each individual as he or she talked. The people on the tapes led normal lives, were average on psychological tests, and had no symptoms, according to Drummond.

The results are frightening, but far from unexpected.

"Forty percent of the psychiatrists chose 'acute paranoid schizophrenia' to describe these examples of normal verbal behavior," Drummond reports in *Mother Jones.* "One result of the study was particularly upsetting: the more experienced the psychiatrist, the more likely he or she was to choose a more pathological diagnosis."

(Even *more* upsetting is the fact that the physicians, including psychiatrists, who remain as full-time VA doctors are the same older, "more experienced" ones noted by Drummond. Those physicians who do leave the agency generally do so by age forty.)

Once a veteran is diagnosed, therapy begins, and therapy often —in the VA, almost always—includes prescribing pills. The choice of medication is virtually a foregone conclusion: Valium or Thorazine.

The VA is proud of its position in the race to prescribe more and stronger pills, tablets, and liquid medication for its patients. It preens in its February 1977 report, *The most frequently occurring diagnoses in VA hospitals—1971–1976,* "The extensive use of antipsychotic drugs [drug companies have brainwashed the medical community into dropping the less graphic word tranquilizer] has contributed greatly to reducing the number of hospitalized patients and in shifting the focus of treatment of mental illness from institutional care to community-based outpatient treatment programs."

That statement is true as far as it goes. The VA has, indeed, established a network of out-patient mental hygiene facilities, and the annual rate of discharge increased from 4.97 per bed in 1971 to 13.08 in 1976. Implicit in all that, the VA would have you believe, is that the "cure" rate has also increased, thereby establishing the efficacy of drug treatment and the progressive attitude the VA has toward its psychiatric charges.

But, in fact, that perception is erroneous. The massive doses of drugs do nothing to improve the emotional status of the patient, even under the best medicating and prescribing procedures.

Reports in the authoritative *Archives of General Psychiatry* in 1974 show that, yes, there are fewer hospitalizations for patients taking tranquilizers but, no, there is little or no improvement in social and interpersonal functioning outside the hospital. "People on tranquilizers merely care less about their delusions," explains Dr. Drummond. "Unfortunately, they care less about other things, too."

Drummond refers to another study, sponsored by the National Institute of Mental Health, which demonstrated that tranquilizers did little or nothing to mitigate the problems of chronic schizophrenics—a large percentage of patients. "The drugs served only to shorten the duration of acute psychoses and reduce the frequency of rehospitalization due to relapses," he notes. "They did nothing for social alienation or blunted emotions."

The sad irony of those findings, and the blatant insensitivity they reveal, are nowhere more manifest than in the horrors rampaging through the VA's 692-bed medical center in San Juan, Puerto Rico. There, as a congressional committee discovered to its dismay, the VA's free-handed dispensing of a major tranquilizer, Valium, has turned the affected veteran population into a significant addict community second in numbers only to those abusing the illicit narcotic heroin.

"The VA in Puerto Rico seems to be contributing to drug problems and then treating the problem they created," reports the House Select Committee on Narcotics Abuse and Control on its 1979 fact-finding mission to the Caribbean. What the committee, headed by former Rep. Lester Wolff (D.-N.Y.), learned in two days of hearings was mind-boggling.

To begin with, the VA was unable to provide the Congress members with reliable figures on the numbers of veterans actually participating in the different treatment programs. Once that was sorted out, the committee found the San Juan VA to be "the single biggest source for the diversion of illicit drugs used in conjunction with methadone," even though the VA does not have a methadone treatment program in Puerto Rico.

Instead, the VA sends the methadone to veterans ostensibly enrolled in programs run by the Commonwealth. The methadone, which blocks heroin craving but creates its own addiction, is then sold on the streets at a healthy profit. Mailing the prescriptions to "these correspondence school" patients is "irresponsible" and "shocking," the committee notes. How many veterans are involved is not clear. The VA testified only 192 were participating. Commonwealth figures, which the committee considered to be more accurate, were 1,239 for 1978 and 840 for 1979.

In its drug dependency program, in which Vietnam veterans are the main clients, "fifty percent . . . had been abusing heroin while forty percent entered the program with Valium as their primary drug of abuse." The Valium that addicted these veterans was issued by the San Juan VA pharmacy. The prescriptions were ordered by VA doctors. Puerto Rico's VA, not surprisingly, has the highest per-capita patient intake per year for any hospital in the entire VA system.

To add to the VA-induced epidemic, doctors at the hospital prescribe routinely as many as three drugs at one time, including Valium and Librium. This "polypharmacy," as the medical profession bizarrely refers to it, resulted in the distribution of 13 million doses of psychoactive drugs in 1978.

In that year, VA physicians wrote scripts for an incredible 346,000 doses of 200-milligram Thorazine, 134,810 doses of 10-milligram Librium, 426,000 doses of 25-milligram Librium, 2,700 doses of 100-milligram Librium, and a whopping 3,089,440 doses of Darvon (since found to have serious side effects).

Frequently, the client never gets to use this medicinal largesse. With drugs like Percodan selling wholesale on the street at $6.70 for one hundred tablets and Ritalin going for $10 for one hundred 20-milligram tabs, the overdosed vet prefers the tidy profit to a blissed-out zombie state. "The Veterans Administration hospital in Puerto Rico, after having prescribed 1,939,488 doses of either 65-milligram or 100-milligram Darvon, told the committee that there was a significant problem with Darvon," the committee report notes drily.

The VA does not recognize a drug disability per se, since the agency's regulations prohibit compensation for willful abuse of drugs. "Most of our patients are compensated for having a neuropsychiatric disorder even though the major symptom is drug-related," the hospital's director told the committee. The committee was also informed by United States Drug Enforcement Agency

personnel that the VA has openly stated that the prescribing policies were intended "to make zombies of these guys so they would
not cause any trouble." In all, 20,000 patients received at least one
prescription in 1978; 18,000 of them got their 59,000 prescriptions
(two million dosage units) via the U.S. mail.

The perpetuation of control over the needful patient that the
charade encourages was strikingly illustrated by the testimony of
Dr. Perez Cruet, the hospital's chief of psychiatry. He acknowledged to the committee that unless a patient agreed voluntarily to
undergo a urine analysis, there was no way to distinguish between signs of psychosis and a drug-related problem! In other
words, veterans with a drug problem might be given prescribed
drugs for psychiatric problems that may in fact be drug or poly-
drug problems. The spectacle of a veteran being prescribed, say,
Valium, when his problem is Valium addiction, is beyond the
bounds of even the VA's usual three-ring mentality.

If that weren't injustice enough, federal investigators uncovered fraud in the midst of negligence—"a variety of embarrassments for the Veterans Administration," is the way the committee
put it.

A General Accounting Office (GAO) report in 1978 revealed the
fact determined by VA investigators that one psychiatrist had
billed the VA for $9,785 in a one-month period. The billing, from
a non-VA doctor hired on a per-patient basis, includes services
rendered on Sunday, September 8, 1974, for thirty-three fifty-
minute sessions—a total of twenty-seven and a half hours for the
one day.

The VA paid the man with no questions asked.

The GAO report also disclosed that seven full-time VA psychiatrists were treating veterans on a fee basis, something strictly
forbidden by VA regulations, not to mention by basic ethics. Also,
one private psychiatrist, on contract to the VA, was found to be
billing the VA for services never given. And six other psychiatrists saw their patients only a few minutes a week but billed the
VA for the full sessions.

No wonder psychiatrists did little more than hand out pills at
the hospital. They were too busy mailing out fraudulent bills.

Indeed, that's exactly what veterans testified. "The 'too busy to care' attitude of psychiatrists may account for the liberal prescriptions of Darvon, Valium, Librium, and Thorazine," the committee concludes.

As a result of the investigation, nine part-time and full-time physicians were terminated and four others were reprimanded or admonished. A total of $13,435 was recovered from two of the doctors. The VA makes no mention of any restitution, or apologies, offered the patients involved.

In its defense, the VA explained that its prescribing practices were not irresponsible and claimed its drugs would create addiction in "only" seventy-seven "primarily psychologically dependent" (presumably urine-tested) veterans.

Dr. Cruet, the psychiatry chief, in a spasm of bureaucratic double-talk that amazed even the Congress members present, testified that admission criteria require the veteran to enter the program voluntarily so he could be helped to cope with problems such as "risk of frequent hospitalizations, involvement in anti-social activities, marriage breakdowns, prolonged family malfunctioning, and other personal and social maladies to diminish the negative impact or overcome these problematic areas." The program's goals, he said, were to eliminate "the non-prescribed use of drugs."

The committee, calling the goals "noble," questioned the "adequacy" of the efforts. "I strongly believe the VA has contributed to this [drug] problem," asserts former Representative Wolff. "Whenever there are prescriptions by mail, you have a ready avenue for all kinds of misuses of the pills. There is also insufficient examination made of the individual in the outpatient department to determine whether this type of treatment is necessary."

Wolff, who calls himself "a hawk when it comes to drug abuse," says the problems uncovered in Puerto Rico are "very widespread" throughout the system. "The point is, these veterans acquired the habit while in service in Vietnam, and we've never had enough drug treatment centers to help them."

Referring to the fact that 65 percent of those admitted to the

San Juan VA drug program are Vietnam veterans even though only 27.3 percent of the total Puerto Rico veteran population served in Vietnam, a staggering statistic, Wolff adds, "I feel very strongly that the young drug abusers are really victims."

The situation in Puerto Rico is doubly compelling, for it puts into sharp focus a community of veterans who also happen to live in a context which itself is discarded and abused. Puerto Rico, the alleged beneficiary of Roosevelt's and Truman's Operation Bootstrap ballyhoo, has an official unemployment rate of over 20 percent. Unofficially, and probably more accurately, the rate is put as high as 50 percent. In addition, 70 percent of the population live below the poverty level and the same number are eligible for food stamps. Sixty-nine percent of those in the island's drug treatment programs—such as they are—are unemployed.

Of all youths in Puerto Rico between the ages of sixteen and twenty-four, 192,000, 36 percent, are out of school and out of work. As if it wasn't obvious enough, the committee reports that it was told "there was a high correlation between unemployment and the recurrence of problems among young people including drug abuse problems." And, it might add, "psychiatric" problems. According to the GAO, 48 percent of the Commonwealth's 19,000 service-connected veterans have received their disability rating for mental disorders.

"These problems," the committee heard the island's Department of Social Services testify, "are attributed to the clash between rising expectations and immediate realities of poverty and unemployment." Something one does not need a urine analysis to measure.

Not coincidentally, Puerto Rico, awash in helplessness, was also one of the human laboratory sites used for the original experimental testing of blood-clotting birth control pills—as well as the early research done to evaluate the effects of those promising new tranquilizer drugs before they were released, their deleterious kinks ironed out of them, to the general public. With those kinds of precedents, one can hardly fault the veteran who acts on the realization that the "mentally disabled" label can raise his monthly compensation payments from $240 a month at 50 percent physical disability to $800–$1,000 monthly for a 100 percent ser-vice-connected psychiatric disability. The game of diagnosis has come full circle, and everyone benefits—the pill companies, the VA budgeteers, the psychiatrists mainlining federal cash, the ad-dicts on the street, the veteran.

Except that the slag-heaped veteran, foraging through the shambles of a disinterested, venal bureaucracy in order to stay alive, carries the "crazy" stigma around with him forever.

Like Alice in Wonderland, the veteran hospitalized at a VA medical center must learn to contend with a world that is, if not perverse, at least turned inside out. Unlike the fictional Alice, however, the sick or disabled vet quickly discovers it is not a dream that has distorted his or her reality.

The looking-glass effect, in fact, starts on admission. For some, like Edwin Zamora, it doesn't end until three weeks after the last 100-milligram Thorazine tablet has been sweated, urinated, or vomited out of the body.

Zamora, who had once worked at the western VA facility in which he was hospitalized in September 1975 after complaining of severe headaches, was required to sign a statement that he would not drink alcohol or use unprescribed drugs during his stay at the facility. If the agreement was broken, the fine print read, "My Treatment Team will take the appropriate action and that immediate discharge, commitment or locked ward may be the action taken." In addition, refusal to submit to alcohol- or drug-detection tests would *automatically* "indicate that I have been using alcohol or non-prescribed drugs."

A growing body of legal literature and court decisions now exists to protect the hospitalized patient from being coerced into submitting to administrative decrees that would be considered violations of civil and due-process rights anywhere else, even disregarding the suspect therapeutic value such arbitrary unilat-eral contracts possess. A bit before his time, Zamora took his own self-protective action. Against doctors' orders, he stopped taking the tranquilizers, which he felt were at least partially responsible for his problems.

And he left the hospital without the written consent of those charged with his care.

"They weren't doing me any good there. I played pool a lot. I asked them to let me work on the hospital grounds, yard work, simple things like that. They told me I wasn't even well enough to roll a ball of tape," adds Zamora, thirty-four, a licensed practical nurse. "But they never put that in my records.

"They never listened to me when I told them the medication was bothering me. I was going around like a zombie. I threw them [the pills] away. It took me three weeks to a month to get myself together, to detoxify myself from that. To this day, I'm not ashamed. I was sick, I guess. But instead of taking me to the medical ward for my headaches, they treated me as a crazy guy.

"I'm not putting down the VA. It's a good hospital. Maybe it was a mistaken diagnosis. But the fact is, I volunteered to be helped. I wanted to get healed, to get cured. When I went there and saw I wasn't getting any help, I said, 'Aw, forget it.' To this day, I still don't know what caused the headaches, and no one ever called me to find out how I was doing."

Zamora has worked steadily at a decent job since leaving the hospital three years ago. But he cannot get back his Civil Service position at the VA, where he was doing well. He receives an annuity, in effect a forced retirement, a situation that bothers him deeply.

As does his brief experience as a patient.

"After I was given all those drugs, I started to drink coffee—it kept me semi-alert. Otherwise, if I had just kept on with the medication, I don't know where I'd be today. They said I was depressed. Who wouldn't be when they start telling you that you won't be able to return to work, that you won't be able to support your family? The drugs made me shake violently. If you saw me then, you'd say this man must be out of his mind. When I told them the medication was bothering me, they switched me to another drug.

"You can't rock the boat when you're in the system. They call you crazy or a rebel. They don't believe your stories, anyway."

Some help, however, may be on the way in the form of a court-ordered mandate. A decision handed down in 1979 by U.S. District

Court Judge Joseph L. Tauro in Boston affirms the psychiatric patient's constitutional rights to have a say in his or her treatment, including the right to reject drugs prescribed by the doctor. Tauro's ruling in the class-action suit states, in part, "Although committed mental patients do suffer at least some impairment of their relationship to reality, most are able to appreciate the benefits, risks and discomfort that may reasonably be expected from receiving psychotropic medication."

He ordered the Boston State Hospital staff to end the forced use by patients of such drugs as Thorazine, Valium, Mellaril, and Haldol. Presumably that decision will also affect the VA's treatment agreements, which veterans like Ed Zamora have been forced to sign.

Even the VA's own research indirectly lends support to a move in that direction. A team of scientists at the Coatesville, Pennsylvania, VA hospital has reported that not only can long-term drug use lead to psychiatric disorders, but that an individual's choice of drugs may determine the illness he develops. The researchers, on the faculty of the University of Pennsylvania, caution against making too much of these early results. But the relevant findings here are associated with the patients who ranked high on general pathology and depression scales, including five who tried to kill themselves. What these veterans all had in common was the prolonged overuse of depressant drugs. Among them are Valium and Librium.

The VA, of course, has not been unaware of the in-hospital excesses. It just chooses to ignore them.

The 1977 National Academy of Sciences study notes, for example, that 15.7 percent of the tranquilizing drugs in effect at the time of their evaluation were above the recommended dosages and that 20 percent of all psychotic patients were getting two or more of the drugs. In all, the team wrote, "it is evident that, in prescribing and administering drugs to psychiatric patients, the observed practices in VA hospitals are at variance with the VA's own policies and guidelines concerning polypharmacy and recommended dosages."

Elsewhere, NAS cites a report to the Administrative Conference of the United States that suggests that approximately 25 percent of VA psychiatric patients are committed involuntarily and that "the VA's admission and release procedures were inadequate to meet the legal rights of those patients and, perhaps, their treatment needs as well."

NAS concludes that policies regarding drug prescriptions and use need "urgent correction."

In response, the VA has had a series of postgraduate training seminars. "The situation has greatly improved," says Dr. Jack Ewalt, director of the VA's Mental Health and Behavioral Sciences Service. "But I would like to see it get better."

"This is a difficult problem all over in medicine," says Dr. Julian David, a psychiatrist and chief of staff at Murfreesboro. "There is a psychological component to every medical condition. I don't care if it's a pain in the finger."

David feels that doctors would rather stay away from invoking the tools of psychiatry, if at all possible. "They're not looking to refer this one or that one," he says. "If something does crop up and they're not tuned in to psychiatry properly—they don't have enough background and training—then they tend to push the button: 'Get him outta here. Call the psychiatrist. The guy is a nut.' Whereas somebody else who has some background would tend to say, 'What's the matter?' and so forth."

David suggests the situation has to be dealt with from both the side of the patient as well as that of the staff. "If the patient is acting up—he did something, it's true—but the reactions of the staff got him more stirred up. It wasn't handled properly. So when you go on the ward for a consultation, it's an educative process for the patient as well as for the staff."

Medications, David adds, frame a similar picture. "It's not uncommon. And not only at the VA. It's at all hospital systems: chemical restraints, get 'em quiet, let's have a nice peaceful place here. But if you don't need to shoot a fly with a cannon, why do that? In many instances, you don't need this tremendous cannon full of all kinds of pills and everything to knock a guy out and keep him like a zombie. Depending on the other therapeutic avenues that you have, then your use of medication could be less.

"There is such a thing as dulling a patient to the point where they can't even perceive an acute appendicitis. And, of course, this is tragic. So, it's not just that you have zombies walking around who can't really relate that much, and everything's nice and peaceful. You can be doing something to their physical being that is masking certain things. We don't do that here. I feel strongly about that."

Edwin Zamora feels strongly, too. With his head cleared of the drug-induced fog and his body rid of the toxic chemicals, he is putting his life back in order, without the interference of the VA.

"As far as I'm concerned, I'm okay," he says. "As far as they're concerned—I don't know."

Staff Writing Letters to Newspapers: Staff are ad-
vised and cautioned about writing letters to newspapers concerning problems within the hospital.
Articles are frequently misinterpreted. There are
other alternatives of solving problems within the
hospital.

                —From Albuquerque VA staff weekly
                newsletter

9

ONE HOSPITAL'S STORY

"I was a perfect specimen of humanity when I went into the
Marine Corps," says Robert Byrd, a World War II veteran
wounded on Guadalcanal January 11, 1943, "three hours after my
sixteenth birthday."

"But now I can't even run anymore. The bottom of my left foot
is numb as hell. There's pain in my right heel and the pain travels
up the leg and keeps me awake at night. Lots of time there's a lot
of pain at the bottom of my spine. It gets discouraging. You go out
there [to the VA], they don't find anything, and they give you a
bunch of pills to take. I've had Darvon, Librium, and aspirin from
the VA for years. But there's no solution, and when they do find
out what's wrong with me, they say it's congenital."

Byrd's VA medical records suggest he has become the victim
of the most amazing coincidence of all time. Blasted by a high-
explosive bomb in combat against the Japanese, the fifty-two-
year-old former plumber and steamfitter has been told by the VA
that the disabling injury, which has necessitated extensive surgery, was actually present at birth.

238

No prior medical exam, including his Marine Corps physical, indicated such a congenital condition. Yet the VA insists he was born with a serious physical defect in the same area of his body that was hit with a military explosion. "The VA conveniently overlooked that wound in the middle of my back for twenty years," Byrd says. "All I wanted was fifty or sixty percent disability. I figure they owe me for thirty years anyway."

Byrd, unemployed because of his condition, now receives 40 percent disability compensation, all related to muscle damage, not to the spine itself. Like many others who have run into a stone wall in pursuit of their rights from the VA, Byrd has been forced to become an expert in all matters surrounding his disability.

He has turned his spacious den-study into a warehouse of documents supporting his position. On one table a thick stack of eight-and-a-half-by-eleven x-ray negatives lies next to one of the expensive medical texts he has purchased. Folders with hospital and doctor records fill the drawers of several file cabinets. Tucked away in the bottom of one of the storage spaces is a neatly folded white and orange Japanese flag. It is bloodstained. Nearby, a handmade sword hangs from the wall. It once belonged to an officer in the Emperor's army.

"The son of a bitch tried to lop my head off," recalls Byrd, who continued to fight in three campaigns after being wounded. "I shot him."

Byrd's battle with the VA hasn't been as easy.

"Years ago," he says, "it was all over my head. I didn't know what they were talking about. Now, they don't like to talk to me because I do know what I'm talking about."

The evidence, ignored by the VA, bears him out. In fact, current medical literature is clear in confirming that spondylolysis, which the VA claims is Byrd's problem, is basically little more than an outdated theoretical assertion. Byrd insists the proper diagnosis is a fracture of a part of the spine called the pars interarticularis. His private physicians support his position. They are also extremely critical of the VA's handling of the case, both administratively and medically.

"[Mr. Byrd] ... again presented me with a voluminous file from the Veterans Administration, including numerous misquotes regarding previous correspondence, copies of which I have in his records," Byrd's orthopedist wrote in a "To whom it may concern" letter dated April 1, 1975. "I am amazed at the monumental misuse of the English language. In several phrases, I am quoted [by the VA] as using the word 'congenital,' and in review of my records, I am unable to find any such word in relation to the demonstrated defect in the pars interarticularis which has been demonstrated by x-ray.

"The defect which is now seen may very possibly be a result of a fracture. . . . In my opinion, this is related to the rather extensive injury which he suffered during World War II at the age of 16."

On January 22, 1975, another private orthopedic specialist wrote that "it has repeatedly been proven that spondylolysis can develop later in life as a result of stress . . . and it is not necessarily of congenital origin. . . . [I]n all probability . . . this is an acquired condition following his injury. . . . It is felt that this condition is service-connected."

For the careful, conservative medical profession, those statements are about as close as you can get to a definitive positive diagnosis.

Byrd's problems took a bizarre turn fifteen years ago when he was admitted to the Albuquerque VA for the operation on his spine. Byrd, the 1965 "Optimist of the Year" for his work with Boy Scouts, entered the hospital with what he was told was a 100 percent service-connected disability. After the surgery, "I was told the injury was congenital and I was no longer service-connected for it." He left the hospital in a body cast and returned home to enormous bills and a foreclosure notice and lien on his property.

"I lost everything except my car," he says. Byrd is a chunky, moon-faced man with wavy hair who moves slowly because of the pain wracking the lower part of his body. Surrounding him on the walls of his den are a cluster of scouting awards just to the left of a large color map of the world. Above the map is a gold-painted replica of a fierce eagle in flight.

A color photo of the young marine in full dress uniform is

placed directly under three oiled hunting rifles. Byrd, who enlisted at age fifteen after he had learned his brother was taken
prisoner of war on Wake Island, says he has never used the fire-
arms because of his injury. Folded tidily under a coffee table is an
American flag, its blue field and white stars facing up, according
to regulations.

"If it hadn't been for a lot of good people in Albuquerque, my
family would have starved to death," he says. "I hate those bas-
tards over that, and that's why I'll never change my opinion about
them.

"I've never asked anybody for help, except what I felt was
coming to me from the VA. When you enlist you feel you are
entitled to be taken care of by your country for service you've
given to your country. I haven't worked since that operation, and
the numbness has only come since the surgery. It wasn't there
before."

Byrd is still actively pursuing his case. "I'm not totally against
the VA," he tells anyone who will listen, "but I do think the vet is
entitled to good care."

"The most sobering experience I've ever had was with a fellow, a patient, who sat there while I asked for his record," Dr.
Gerald Parkes remembers. "Eventually it came. I complained
about this time after time, the delay in records coming back to the
patient.

"When it came, I opened the folder and the first thing you saw
was his death certificate. And I looked at him and I said to myself,
'There are certain people who are suspicious. There are certain
people who are suspicious, sure, and they don't like to see their
death certificate.' I sort of fumbled around, then slammed the
cover shut before he could see his goddamn death certificate.
That, I would say, is the state of records in the VA. I have never
seen in all my life worse records than at the VA.

"Eventually, they get them sorted out. But in the meanwhile
it's time-consuming."

Gerald Parkes chuckles softly and incredulously at the recol-
lection. For six years, Parkes, a general practitioner with a mas-

ter's degree in public health from Harvard, took note of the antics passed off as medical care at the Albuquerque VA.

In 1977, fed up, he quit.

The Albuquerque VA Medical Center is almost as old as the VA itself. Built in 1932 as a tuberculosis hospital, it has grown to a modern general medical and surgical facility. Along the way, it acquired that mark of VA respectability—a medical school affiliation. Although it is one of the older facilities in the system, it maintains a cared-for physical appearance on the outside. Set on a lovely knoll on the southern edge of an expanding city, the cluster of more than twenty-five buildings, architecturally in keeping with the adobe-pueblo style of the region, overlooks Albuquerque and the ever-changing Sandia Mountains to the east.

The long driveway starting at the guardhouse at the main gate takes the visitor up a slight incline past green manicured lawns. New trash cans are strategically placed, and giant shade trees, precious in the New Mexico sunshine, provide ample sitting areas for patients and their guests. The rolling grounds comprise the lushest, best-kept hospital campus in the city.

It is a pleasant place to be ill—until you enter the wards. Devoid of air-conditioning, except in administrative suites and doctors' offices, the atmosphere is one of dusty-dry harried resignation. Overworked nurses try to complete routine chores while technicians who ask for better working conditions are reminded of the new thirty-dollar-a-roll wallpaper gracing the stairwell walls. Rumor has it that doctors, hassled by the sheer numbers of patients they must see, frequently "misplace" charts under a pile of paperwork or in a bottom drawer so as to postpone the incessant demands of record-keeping.

Farther into the hospital, on Ward 5, terminal and long-term patients are subjected to hundred-degree-plus temperatures in the summer, four beds to a room, bare walls, and spare furnishings. A few feet away, the rooms are light and airy, where the patients with more optimistic prognoses have their own recreation room. It is a place, too, where ambulance drivers dread the sight of the emergency room late at night. "The VA is the bottom of the barrel. It's the worst hospital in town," declares an experienced employee of Albuquerque Ambulance Service who has brought patients to every health-care facility in the city. "You drive in with some poor bleeding sucker and all the clerk is interested in is the last four digits of his Social Security number. I always write up a report on what goes on there, but I get nowhere. It's real bad."

On Ward 2-E, a young Vietnam veteran lies attached to life-giving machines, unmoving, semiconscious. He was operated on in 1971—a relatively simple procedure—and something went terribly wrong. During the operation, the surgeon told the anesthesiologist to turn off the gas. He turned off the oxygen instead. The out-of-court settlement provided for complete medical (custodial) care for the rest of his life and a sum of money reportedly in six figures.

The veteran's mother visits every day and on occasion has complained to the administration about dirt on the floor.

Down the newly painted hall, past the freshly hung curtains that block the hot-air ducts, an elevator stops, letting off a trio of orthopedic residents. An in-house sign, one of those clever stick-figure public relations morale boosters that give employees the illusion of participating in management decisions, hangs from the lift's rear wall. It reads, "Don't just knock what's bad—suggest something better."

Several have tried.

"The filth is what I couldn't tolerate," explains Mrs. Billie Jean Corcoran, "so I made sure I brought some Dutch Cleanser and a razor blade to clean up. I wouldn't put an animal in the tub they used."

Mrs. Corcoran has an extended familiarity with the Albuquerque VA. From 1954 to 1975, her husband, Edward, was in and out of the facility. In 1975, frustrated and angered by the treatment he was receiving, Billie Jean Corcoran hired a private R.N. to attend to him at home. The VA sent over an aide two days a week.

"I couldn't just leave anyone with him," she says. "I usually came up with what was wrong with my husband long before they did."

Corcoran, in the navy in Okinawa during World War II and

chief engineer for the New Mexico state plumbing board, was 100 percent service-connected for multiple sclerosis. "He's been on every floor over there. They weren't concerned about my husband, period," she says flatly. "They'd forget to give him his Dilantin. So I had to slip him his medicine. They sometimes let him go so long without it, I thought he'd never come home. It was up to me to make sure he got it.

"If he didn't get it, he wouldn't come out of his seizures, and he would die."

Which is exactly what happened.

Brought to the hospital because of an emergency—the only reason Mrs. Corcoran would allow him anywhere near the place —Edward Corcoran died March 15, 1978, at the age of sixty-one.

Someone, she says, forgot to give him his Dilantin.

"My husband dreaded going over there. He always said they treated him like a guinea pig. I wouldn't go there again, and I'm really sorry I brought my husband there."

Mrs. Corcoran, a native Albuquerquean who now spends a lot of time with her daughter and granddaughter, also recalls the problems they encountered with the drugs prescribed by the VA. "They'd send us Valium and Percodan, and a lot of them were missing. We finally had to count the pills to make sure we got what was written on the label."

The experience has even modified her attitudes toward an impatient younger generation.

"A lot of times at the hospital I'd see Vietnam veterans waiting around. I've actually watched them throw their files. They weren't getting anything from throwing their files, but they were there from nine in the morning to five in the evening, and the doctor didn't see them. How would you feel?"

Waiting for help—help both morally and legally mandated— was not confined to Vietnam soldiers. Multiple sclerosis victims and their families are an energetic, tight-knit, aggressive group in Albuquerque, and elsewhere. The focus of a great deal of their attention is on the VA hospital, particularly the prosthetics department, which is responsible for providing physical aids and sensory devices to veterans eligible for them.

It may be because Albuquerque is so poorly run that the VA central office in Washington felt obliged to intervene in its operation. Max Cleland, who claims a special interest in rehabilitative medicine, sent a personal emissary, outside of normal VA channels, to New Mexico to examine the situation. When he arrived, Nathan Nolan, a former rehabilitation director for the state of Georgia, refused to acknowledge the purpose of his mission. He also refused to talk to veterans who had complaints.

"Nolan told me, 'What can I do for you, Tony?' recalls Tony Gonzales, the Vietnam infantryman forced by VA inaction to wait ten months for a leg brace only to wind up with a fifteen-day commitment to the psychiatric ward. "I said he could get things straightened out at the hospital. He said to me, 'No, what can I do for *you?'* He kept asking me what would make me happy. It seems like they're willing to do anything for me now. I think it's to keep me from bitching, which I won't stop anyway."

Gonzales took another vet, Jack Scratton, to the meeting with Nolan. "He had complaints, too. I figured if he [Nolan] wanted to hear about conditions here, he'd be interested in hearing about them from someone else, too. But he just ignored Jack. And he made no promises."

"What was once a fine hospital medically has deteriorated as far as patient care is concerned," says Mrs. Maggie Amacker, long after Nolan slipped out of Albuquerque. Amacker's husband, Danny, a World War II veteran of the China and Burma campaigns and formerly a singer and master of ceremonies in the Catskills, is 100 percent service-connected for multiple sclerosis. Danny Amacker goes regularly to the county hospital MS clinic. He has also taken out extra insurance so he can afford another hospital. In addition, the Amackers are paying for physical and occupational therapy at the privately run Rehabilitation Center —all services due him from the VA.

"He just won't go in, even for a checkup," Maggie Amacker, also a former entertainer, says. "Everyone's on an economy binge, saving money, saving public funds. Should it be spent on trees or to provide care? To decorate administrative offices or should it be spent on patients' equipment? I just think it's outrageous."

So did the FBI. On February 8, 1978, federal agents in Albuquerque arrested Larry Weaver at his office in Building One of the medical center. Weaver, who had worked at seven VA hospitals in his fourteen-year Civil Service career, was the chief of Fiscal Service at the time.

He was also committing fraud. Almost $18,000 worth.

Late one night in September 1977, working overtime, Weaver, distraught by the treatment he was getting from his superiors, filed a fraudulent voucher "for payment for certain trees in the amount of $17,640 . . . [for] approximately one-hundred trees to be delivered to the Veterans Administration Hospital, by Lashlee Landscaping Company, a non-existent business entity . . . ," reads the one count he was convicted on in the indictment.

Weaver's larcenous activity gives a revealing glimpse into the hospital's, and the VA's, operations, and the prevailing pressures that ultimately bubble up to affect patient care.

Weaver's court-mandated psychological report describes his VA employment as "stressful." It goes on,

When he arrived at the hospital in September, 1974, Weaver found that the hospital had a budget deficit of approximately one million dollars. He . . . worked with staff to reduce spending. When he left the hospital, Weaver stated that his staff of twenty were frequently working long hours processing 6,000 vouchers per month. . . . Ultimately, Weaver had responsibility for a 22 million dollar yearly budget.

In January 1977, he lost his assistant in the budget office and personal problems increased at home. The report continues,

His work deteriorated, and when working late one night . . . Weaver stated that he said to himself, 'To heck with it,' and filed a fraudulent voucher. Weaver added that after learning about the investigation, he called the Federal Bureau of Investigation and offered to cooperate.

Further insight is provided by the Classification Summary written by Wiley F. Ward, senior case manager.

Upon arrival in Albuquerque, he [Weaver] states that he found very poor fiscal management and ran into conflicts with his supervisors in an attempt to control this. As a result of these conflicts, he was given a very poor efficiency rating by his supervisor, which hurt his career badly.

Previous to that rating, Weaver had ranked among the top 5 percent of the VA's financial managers. Slotted at a score of 23 percent by his Albuquerque superiors, he dropped precipitously to the bottom of the heap. "The director [when Weaver arrived] had been operating out of his hip pocket for ten years. That's why there was no air-conditioning, that's why nothing was done. He did what he pleased," says a former employee intimately knowledgeable about the affair. "You can't operate a budget that way. The VA finally retired him to Sun City [an Arizona retirement village]."

Instructive also is the way Weaver's misdeed was uncovered. The VA brags about all its committees and teams entrusted with the overseeing of the operations of individual hospitals, but the VA facility had not had a full-scale audit in more than two decades. It was left to a low-level, underpaid secretary, suspicious because the procedure used by Weaver was irregular, to blow the whistle. She discovered it easily enough: Checking the Lincoln, Nebraska, phone book, the purported home of the fictional landscaping company, she quickly learned the firm did not exist.

Weaver was fined $10,000 and sentenced to five years, reduced to two, at the La Tuna federal correctional facility at Anthony, Texas, a place notorious for occasional outbreaks of food poisoning among the inmates. Paroled after serving approximately a year of his term, Weaver is now making a new life for himself in a small town in the South. Weaver took with him, with the blessing of the same government he tried to cheat out of $18,000, a medical retirement check of $800 a month, down somewhat from the $2,373.10 monthly he was receiving at the time of his arrest. The medical retirement was assured when it was suggested by VA officials that he be psychiatrically examined after his arrest but before the trial or sentencing. A little gift from his former employer.

Actually, there were other gifts.

At the time of his landscaping escapade, Weaver was also raising quail, some 4,500 of them. And he was keeping them in the basement of the home he was renting on the hospital's grounds. "Weaver's hope in this . . . venture," states the official report, "was to make between 50 and 100 thousand dollars a year in ultimately selling the quail to retail grocery stores."

Observers familiar with the birds say they were so dirty and smelly that VA maintenance workers balked at cleaning, fumigating and repainting the house at taxpayers' expense after Weaver was sent to other, less hospitable government accommodations. They suggest also that Weaver had already started providing home-raised fowl for a local restaurant. "He was selling quail to private institutions," says a nineteen-year VA employee who finally quit in disgust with the administration of the facility. "One was in Estancia, another was a fried-chicken place in Albuquerque.

"The house was so filthy when Weaver left, they had to use hospital ground crews to clean up the quail crap. It was piled so high, they had to use shovels."

In fact, the remaining odor was so persistent and difficult to remove—the house stayed vacant for months afterward—that several coats of paint were needed before workmen could move in and complete the renovation. None of the costs were borne by Weaver.

The FBI showed no interest in this particular use of federal property, although it did recommend that some rabbit cages removed by other employees be returned. The G-men joked with Weaver about the operation, expressed some curiosity about how the birds were raised, but that was all. "It really wasn't anything," said Special Agent Lane DeSilva.

Nor did the FBI investigate the threats Weaver received while in prison.

According to a well-placed source, Weaver got a letter, addressed to him at La Tuna, which strongly suggested it would "not be to your [Weaver's] advantage" to speak to elected officials or other authorities about the landscaping fraud. "It was anonymous, and it made it clear he shouldn't talk," the source says. "I don't know who sent it, or why."

Even when money is not being squandered on trees, fraudulently or otherwise, it is not necessarily being used for the maximum benefit of the patient, despite Maggie Amacker's most fervent wishes. Nowhere is this more evident than in the department that perked the interest of the mysterious Nathan Nolan and brought him on his secret mission to the Duke City.

The former head of the Prosthetics and Sensory Aides service was a forty-seven-year-old, 100 percent disabled and service-connected former motel assistant manager and housekeeping trainee named William Powell. He arrived at his Albuquerque post in late 1973 with only four months of prosthetics training—he should have had twelve according to regulations—and just a year and a half of prosthetics work experience in a small outpatient unit at Muskogee, Oklahoma. With a June 1959 B.S. in business and economics from Central Missouri State, Powell was responsible at Albuquerque for a busy in-patient and outpatient division with a budget of over a quarter of a million dollars for supplies alone.

He was paid well for his efforts. Powell got a VA salary of approximately $23,000, which, in addition to his service-connected compensation of about $2,000 a month, tax-free, put him in an income bracket more than five times that of most of the veterans he was hired to serve.

"He was always pleasant to anyone who had some support behind him," says a former close assistant of his. "But if they were in bad financial straits, he was particularly bad to them. He always took the attitude, 'If I made it, why can't they?' He was a real politician."

On occasion, the VA provided Powell with free psychiatric care, and paid his $1,200 bill for dental work at a private clinic. In addition, his compensation status, which included a partial paralysis of his right side, entitled his two children to an expense-paid college education. Powell quickly and easily took to the outdoor life-style of the Southwest, enjoying, among other pursuits, the golfing and social company of the owners of Highland Pharmacy, a local pharmaceutical supply house.

At work, Powell liked to show how busy his bailiwick was. For instance, the quarterly report sent to the VA central office for the period ending March 31, 1977, lists, for four different categories of disability, a total of 2,116 veterans receiving service. A second set of records, however, reveals that the total for the four categories is actually 1,699—a padding of 20 percent, and a concomitant potential budget increase. The report with the inflated figures, *Cumulative inventory of active prosthetics disabilities—veterans with continuing eligibility,* was signed by William Powell.

"Basically," explains someone who worked closely with him, "he kept inactive cases on active."

There were many patient complaints.

Billie Jean Corcoran, for one, recalls with anger the equipment Powell sent to her dying husband—a disintegrating electric hospital bed held together with bailing wire.

She returned it.

"Powell was upset because I wouldn't take the same bed back," she remembers, looking at the color photos she took of the bed at the time. "He sent me the bed with the wire after I had already returned another one with a broken shaft. I was furious."

The beds were from Highland Pharmacy.

Ultimately, Corcoran forced the hospital's assistant director to get Powell to provide an appropriate piece of equipment.

It was not the first time top administrators at the hospital had heard about Powell's department.

On April 7, 1977, Edward Case, chief, Corrective Therapy section, sent a memorandum to his boss, Dr. Asja Kornfeld, chief, Rehabilitation Medicine service. It concerned the ordering of adapted van equipment for a veteran in a wheelchair who was currently involved in the section's driver-training program. Case outlined the careful evaluation he and an assistant made in formulating their recommendations for an appropriate lift for the patient. After pointing out in the memo an earlier error by Powell in his choice of equipment for another veteran, Case continues,

Mr. Powell has been insistent on ordering a Helper lift rather than a Ricon. He says it is cheaper. He says that a local supplier is willing to send a man to the Helper factory to learn how to install the lift. Mr. Powell says he feels we should be willing to order the Helper because of the local supplier making this commitment.

The real problem, we feel, lies in the basic type of lift the patient requires and not in the brand name. . . . [T]here are a number of other lifts on the market that would fit this patient's needs better than the Helper. . . . Mr. Powell [says] the Helper representative is going to modify the lift for $160 so it can be used [by this patient].

We feel that the Helper lift may pose safety hazards for this particular patient. . . . We feel that the trust and confidence of the patient . . . may be jeopardized if he is not satisfied with the lift system. . . .

We do not . . . feel it appropriate to compromise quality patient care because of obligations to private vendors, professional jealousy [or] brand names. . . .

All of these factors have been discussed with Mr. Powell but he still maintains that he will order the Helper lift.

Six weeks later, Case sent another memo to Dr. Kornfeld. "Since the memorandum of 4/7/77, the following things have occurred," he wrote.

1. The Helper lift was installed on Mr. C.'s 1970 Dodge van. The door actuators could not be modified to fit the van. Highland Pharmacy, who installed the lift, told the patient they would order other actuators for the doors. . . .

3. He also states that Highland Pharmacy offered him a compromise and gave him hand controls. . . . Patient states he is happy with the arrangement and doesn't want to "jeopardize anyone's job over it." He states Mr. Powell approved the compromise arrangement. . . .

4. a. Why was there assurance given that the lift modification could be done for $160 to fit a swinging door van when in reality this is apparently impossible . . . ?

c. Why is the patient concerned about jeopardizing anyone's job since nobody [here] has indicated to him in any way that any controversy was raised concerning his van? It must be assumed he was informed of this by some other source.

On May 19, a day later, Dr. Kornfeld finally acted, sending Case's two memos, along with an attachment of her own, to the acting chief of staff. "I request," she wrote, "that no substitute equipment be issued—after we specifically order what is needed —to avoid similar difficulties and *embarrassment* in the future." [Italics added.]

Less than a month later, hospital administrator Birmingham, in a memorandum to Powell, expressed his "particular concern that a contractor has not delivered what was ordered." Case says that "there have been no problems since that one case. I've had no more difficulties. The equipment I recommend, I get."

"It's pathetic the way Mr. Powell treats some people," says Mrs. Corcoran. "You can go over there one day and he would be perfectly normal. The next time he'd be storming about something. He just isn't a man who should be dealing with crippled people. I'm not condemning him. He's just too ill. Who would send beds that were wired and had broken shafts?

"You know," she continues, "we used to have a very efficient company repairing the equipment. They knew exactly what to do. When Mr. Powell took over, he farmed the work out to three others. Then he dropped the reliable company. And one of the remaining companies kept sending out bad equipment—Highland. I always wondered why he did that."

"Whatever Highland had, he pushed it," says a former VA employee. "Over half of his budget each month went to that place. They're very close friends."

Close enough, apparently, to delay getting help for a patient.

On June 9, 1977, Powell received a prescription from Dr. Kornfeld to order a Ricon lift from Stagewest, another supplier in town. The request, Charge Appropriation 36×0102, Exp. Acct. 3403, was refused by Powell. Less than two months later, after the contract with Stagewest had expired, Powell ordered the same lift from Highland Pharmacy.

William Caley, the ex-owner of the company dropped by Powell, tries to hide his bitterness. "I don't like to point a finger," he says. "To me, if I was entitled to the business, fine. I would never buy my business. We sold wheelchairs to fit the patient, not just to sell a wheelchair. If a person needs a piece of equipment, he's got to have what he needs, not what I've got. If we didn't have it in stock, we'd go and get it. We kept about fifteen thousand dollars in parts in stock. We treated them right. We had a lot of respect for the boys."

Caley agrees with the criticism leveled against Powell and the way he ran his service.

"The vets are right. He doesn't buy the right equipment. I'd offer to go up there, help out, fix some small things—free—but he didn't care to have me hanging around. I didn't want to be where I wasn't wanted."

Caley, in the business for more than sixteen years, questions the present purchasing arrangement. "When I was there, all wheelchairs were bought from GSA [General Services Administration] before Powell arrived. If he's buying them from Highland, he can get himself in trouble with the VA. All that stuff should come from GSA. We just did the repair work."

In addition, he says, Highland may very well be in violation of the law because they are being paid to deliver and pick up beds from the VA. "That's against ICC regulations." Caley is philosophical about it. "One thing people can't say is that I bought the business. I just wasn't a golfer. Never liked to play golf, so I never got the business."

"I feel sorry for him [Powell]," says the wife of a veteran who is immobilized from a stroke after twenty-three years of honorable military service and a term in the state legislature. "But I also feel sorry for the people he's doing in." Her husband, a World War II infantryman who spent six months at the Albuquerque VA in 1971–72 and was "constantly wet in bed from urine because he wasn't being rotated," had been refused equipment and help from Powell. Although she is still trying to get her husband his benefits, she is adamant, almost vicious, about not allowing him back into the hospital.

"Our medical bills are over ten thousand dollars this year. He worked twice as hard as his civilian counterpart because he expected to get his benefits. But we're not getting them. He's given his life for those benefits, and all he gets are doctors and students pricking him and examining him.

"What's his, we want. We feel he's entitled to it. But instead you get a whole lot of runaround—that's it."

Like many others, she is fearful of permitting her name to be used. Her husband, a retired colonel and once-avid outdoorsman, now sits propped up in a large chair, unable to speak. His wife has placed the chair near the large window in their modest trailer-home, facing the majestic Sandia Mountains he once hiked. The only sounds he makes are occasional childlike sobbing noises that come out strangled from the top of his throat.

"My friends keep telling me not to rock the boat," his wife says, "because we might lose the benefits we already have."

She looks over at her husband, who is crying with shallow, irregular heaves.

"But Powell has already done that," she says.

In 1979, William Powell retired from the VA, after a VA audit team from Los Angeles made its first visit to Albuquerque in more than twenty years.

Other things of a much different nature took place several years earlier, when the VA sent a special investigator to Albuquerque to look into alleged extracurricular activities in the morgue and other parts of the hospital. During the latter part of 1969 and for about a year thereafter, the hospital played host to a sort of floating pornographic movie house, complete with grainy films and sweaty palms. Using the morgue and selected office space, employees kicked in a buck apiece weekly for the opportunity to view what the investigator's report says one participant called "a black and white, poor-quality 16-mm. film."

"They showed them in the morgue using VA equipment and personnel, on VA time," recalls the technical supervisor of the histological laboratory, which included the morgue. He and others insist the shows, at least initially, were organized by a physician who headed one of the hospital's technical services. This doctor vigorously denies the accusation.

"They were just doing it for the fun of it, I guess," says the histology lab employee.

Lunch hour was a favorite time for viewing the pictures, and a variety of offices was used. At one showing, according to testimony in the six-page official report, thirty to forty people came by —janitors, technicians, lab technologists, "and various other VA employees." Most of the time, however, less than five showed up for the short viewings. Other testimony suggested that two or three pathology residents were involved in purchasing and showing the movies.

"The films shown in the morgue were primarily about young

children and male sex relations," says the histology supervisor. "Apparently, they kept showing them somewhere else in the hospital after I objected to them being shown in the morgue."

"They were black and white films—one of them showed two women and one man—about ten minutes long," recalls a medical technician who saw them in the medical illustration room. Another lab technician also saw the films in the projection room, and remembers several doctors present.

"I saw some of the movies," the hospital's projectionist acknowledges. "Possibly as many as a half dozen."

After twenty-five years at the Albuquerque VA, he retired before the investigation got under way in 1976 and therefore was never interviewed by the investigators. He says he doesn't remember who was present at the showings. He says he remembers lending his VA projector to somebody, but didn't "necessarily know what they are doing" when equipment was borrowed from him.

"I had a good idea it was going on in my office," he says, adding, "What a guy does on his lunch hour is entirely up to him—smoke, a girl, lunch, drink."

"The films were a minor, tangential issue, a personal matter," say Robert K. Jennings, who was involved in the probe some six years after it all took place. The VA, he notes, first learned of the allegations after coming to Albuquerque to look into unrelated irregularities in one of the laboratories.

Edward Ralowsky, Jr., the special investigator who actually conducted the inquiry, says that there were three people involved in showing the films (only one is acknowledged in the report) and that twenty or twenty-five viewed the pictures at least once, in both the morgue and the medical illustration (projection) room. Viewers included "several doctors, electricians, nurses' aides and technicians.

"I understand you could barely see the figures, the film was so bad."

At the end of the investigation, no disciplinary action was taken against anyone.

"It was a retired employee who showed the films," Ralowsky

says, ignoring the trio theory, and other evidence in the report itself. "He's gone. No films have been shown for a length of time. You can't go back. Time has lapsed. It's unfortunate. It did happen, but it's not going on now. Anyway, we're not out to get an employee in trouble."

Although Ralowsky interviewed several physicians during the course of his investigation, their names were blacked out in the final report. Only those lower in the hierarchy—technicians and such—had their names revealed. Even in pornography, rank has its privileges—in the VA, at least.

For some doctors, however, the rank has lost some of its lustre. As of March 30, 1979, 16.5 percent of the resident physician positions (doctors still in training) in VA Medical Centers were held by foreign medical graduates (FMGs). Nine hospitals were staffed virtually entirely by FMGs in 1978, and thirty-three facilities listed 20 percent or more of their medical doctors as having graduated from a foreign school.

The United States may be a melting pot and the port of huddled masses yearning to breathe free, but when it comes to foreign medical graduates, who also include a small number of American citizens, many veterans and officials would just as soon they went back where they came from.

"My observation is that the VA is attracting many foreign doctors," says Alabama Congress member Bill Nichols, himself a disabled World War II combat veteran. "Number one, I believe a service-connected veteran ought to be able to converse to make his pain and problems known. How can he do that if language is a difficulty?"

The VA, says Dr. Paul East, chief of medical and dental education, is being responsive. For example, it has dramatically reduced the number of FMGs trained at the VA over the past decade, from a high of 32 percent in 1970 to half that amount today. In addition, the VA now has mandatory training in English for those experiencing trouble with the language. But, as Dr. East points out, language is by no means the only barrier the veteran-patient must contend with.

"It may be a problem of acculturation, not one of language," he says. "One patient may perceive a problem, another may not. The medical knowledge of the foreigner who passed [the required medical] tests is adequate to work in a clinical setting. All it comes down to is that there is less likelihood [of] extreme excellence [in the foreign graduate].

"What's left is color, accent, and subtle difference of ethnic background."

"Subtle" may be the wrong word. Try asking the Vietnam vets, like Bobby Muller, who were treated in the VA by doctors from Southeast Asia, or World War II veterans, like Steve Cannizzaro, who were examined by a Japanese physician, or the Albuquerque VA patients who must go through the office of Dr. Wilhelm Ludwig (not his real name).

Sometimes it as subtle as a slap in the face.

"Let's be frank about Dr. Ludwig. Dr. Ludwig was a German officer," says Dr. Gerald Parkes, who was in British intelligence during the war. "We never got along completely well because, I'm sorry, I never got along completely well with German officers. I had seen too much of their goings on.

"How Ludwig made it to this country, and got into such a delicate situation, I don't know."

Dr. Wilhelm Ernst Ludwig is a full-time psychiatrist at the VA Medical Center in Albuquerque, employed as the admitting compensation and pension examiner in the out-patient unit. Unlike most of his colleagues, he has no ties—salary or otherwise—with the affiliated University of New Mexico School of Medicine. Unlike his colleagues, too, he belongs to no medical society or group —not the American Medical Association nationally nor the Albuquerque-Bernalillo County Medical Society locally. Although he proudly talks of attending professional meetings, he is, it would seem, a loner. Or, for some reason, he seems to prefer to keep a low profile.

Some things, however, he is not hesitant to talk about. Once, when a Vietnam veteran came to him complaining of severe pain from shrapnel wounds, Ludwig belittled the discomfort, using himself as an example. "Pain is not so bad," he told the veteran.

"You can make yourself cope with it. During the war I had chest surgery without anesthetic."

Ludwig is sixty-four and the war he referred to is World War II. Born in Gera, Thuringia, in Germany, he was not in the American armed services. Ludwig told the Vietnam veteran that he was a corporal in the German army. He fought many battles against the Communists on the Russian front, he quickly added, and, he offered, he wasn't a Nazi.

In his position in the out-patient clinic, Ludwig makes decisions about compensation eligibility for veterans with emotional problems. At one point, in the early seventies, he raised some hackles among a group of veterans who felt he might have been more sensitive to their needs.

"I couldn't work anymore, my nerves were bothering me, my back was in pain, my whole system was breaking down fast," recalls Robert Garcia, 60, "so I went to the VA."

Garcia is part of a dying breed. He is one of several thousand World War II veterans who spent a debilitating three and a half years in Japanese concentration camps in the South Pacific. Many of them now live in New Mexico, and they have formed the Bataan Veterans Organization to, as one member puts it, "look out for each other."

Ludwig wasn't too enthused when I went to see him in 1973," Garcia continues. "All the POWs had to go see him, and I figured he thought I was just another prisoner of war with a bitch. I tried to tell him about our POW experiences, but he was indifferent, cold. I thought maybe he had seen too many soldiers, too many war injuries. Maybe he wasn't impressed with our POW status. I thought I wasn't the only one being treated that way. I thought, well, maybe it's the way they do things here.

"When you told him something was bothering you, stress, whatever, he said he couldn't see why that would be. I only spent forty-two months as a POW."

Garcia, retired from the Bureau of Revenue and a former hog farmer, finally got his 100-percent disability rating after seeing another doctor. Since then, Ludwig has become much more supportive of the Bataan veterans. "I heard there was a change in him," Garcia, who has a son who is a Vietnam veteran, says. "I don't know what happened. I guess somebody spoke to him. But he's come around to seeing our way of looking at things. For a while, you couldn't get by him."

"He's made a complete change," echoes Leo Padilla, a past president of the Bataan organization. "I don't know why. He used to act like the money was coming out of his pocket."

Ludwig gets livid when the subject is brought up.

"I've shown more insight into the Bataan veterans and I've seen more of them than anyone else," he says, angry that anyone should say otherwise. He says he never heard any complaints, and that, in fact, he attends their functions and gets along with them very well.

"I don't know where you heard that. It's not true."

Earlier in the conversation, he pleasantly discussed, without rancor or defensiveness, his experiences as a German medical student during the war.

Ludwig is physically impressive. He is six feet tall, wiry and strong of build. His heavy black-rimmed glasses accent his hawk-like features. His hair is snow-white. He is alert and aware— clean, stiff, bright, sharp, dogmatic, logical, and precise. He moves crisply down the long hospital corridors, and is deferential to his superiors.

To his patients Ludwig, never certified or formally trained as a psychiatrist, could appear competent but cold. To his colleagues, there were other perceptions.

"We were working in the most awful circumstances where we had people waiting to see the doctor in a little dingy room," Dr. Parkes remembers. "At the same time, we had administration with its carpet and their nice offices and all of that. We had none of this.

"Then, they decided they would spend some money. So, whilst they were spending the money, building a new out-patient area, where did we go? We went into two trailers that were the most disgraceful things I have ever worked in in the whole of my life. I have worked in combat-type conditions. I have worked in Indo-China where we built a hospital in the jungle, and the hospital I built in the jungle was a palace compared with the hospital that they provided at the VA.

"We had two double-wide trailers. They were not even new trailers. They were brought from some national catastrophe, one of those hurricanes [actually, the 1972 Pennsylvania floods]. They brought these wrecked old trailers and shoved them up against the side of the building. They leaked water from the word go. The doors were sliding doors that were falling apart at the hinges. We could not get wheelchairs into the place. We put up with this for the better part of three years.

"I had my office next to Dr. Ludwig, and the walls of this trailer were paper-thin. So, he would holler out things, and my patients would answer his questions. Then he would say, 'Why the hell are you answering that? I didn't ask you that.' Well, it was the guy next door, my patient, answering that, because of the walls.

"The walls were so thin, I'd have to go over to Dr. Ludwig and say, 'Listen, Dr. Ludwig, will you keep quiet?' He'd say [German accent here], 'Vy do you vant me to keep quiet? I am in my own country. I am going to do the right thing.'

" 'No, Dr. Ludwig, it's because your voice is too goddamn loud and they think I'm talking to them.' "

Parkes, a short, animated native of Liverpool now practicing medicine in northern New Mexico, waxes incredulous as he describes Ludwig's medical proclivities.

"His whole diagnosis is made on ethnic probabilities. For example, 'Dr. Ludwig, I have a real problem with this guy and I would like some advice from you as a psychiatrist.' Again, you're stymied, because he isn't a psychiatrist. He never trained as one. So, you'd be asking your colleague, who really wasn't a psychiatrist, his psychiatric opinion. Amazing.

"He would come back with something like, 'Vell, you see, you're dealing with a man who's part Belgian, and he's got some Austrian in him and the Jewish part will go with the Austrian part. . . . You von't be able to treat him that way, but you can do this. . . .'

"I said to myself, 'My God, this guy is strange.' I wanted to know if I should give him [the patient] some Lithium or something else.

" 'Nah, it won't work on him.'

"I listened to this, over and over, through those thin partitions that leaked and I'd hear this weird message of, 'Where did you come from?' and 'What is your ethnic background?'

Another physician who shared a partition with Ludwig in those days, Dr. Diana Kellner, says he was "a conscientious physician, a very careful and thorough history-taker." Ludwig, she says, asked for a patient's ethnic background "only if it was necessary for a psychiatric diagnosis, only when it was relevant to the psychiatric history."

And under what circumstances would that be?

"I don't know, I'm not a psychiatrist," Dr. Kellner said.

Ludwig was born in what is now East Germany on November 27, 1916, where he attended the local Catholic elementary school. After attending the Gymnasium Rutheneum, the equivalent of high school and part of college, he enrolled in the Medizinische Fakultat der Friederich-Schiller-Universitat in Jena, a prestigious medical school just down the road from Buchenwald. Ludwig says he never worked there or in any other concentration camp as a student or doctor.

"I didn't know anything about those things. We worked in civilian hospitals, like BCMC [a local county hospital]."

Training was rigorously controlled while Ludwig was in school.

"The Medical Case," an official Allied document in Volume One of the Nuremberg War Trials:

On paper, medical training under the Nazis differed little from that of the pre-Nazi era. However, its fundamental spirit was ruinously distorted and medical standards suffered a dismal decline.

Medical students had to be 'Aryan,' and were required to belong to the National Socialist Students' League. The students' entire course of studies was constantly interrupted by the demands of the various party organizations to which they were forced to belong. A student whose knowledge of the racial theories and Nuremberg laws was not sufficient would fail his medical examinations.

Particularly deplorable was the degradation of psychiatry. Psychiatric university teaching declined to the level of a mere rehashing of the Nuremberg and sterilization laws. The modern techniques of psychotherapy had been abandoned, and treatment deteriorated to pep talks, admonitions and threats.

The Nazi medical world was flooded with preposterous and wicked notions about superior and inferior races and developed a perverted moral outlook in which cruelty to subjugated races and peoples was praiseworthy. Training in SA and SS formations was hardly calculated to develop physicians who could comprehend even the bare elements of the doctor-patient relationship.

After six years of studies, Ludwig received his diploma on February 28, 1944. It is signed by the Reich Secretary of the Interior. On March 10, he obtained his physician's license from the Thuringia Department of Education. Upon graduation, Ludwig apparently joined the German Army Medical Corps, where he stayed until 1945. From 1946 to 1953 he worked first for the Bavarian Public Health Department and then spent six years in private practice in Polling, a Bavarian hamlet in a resort area twenty-one miles southwest of Munich.

On March 23, 1953, Ludwig was admitted at New York City for permanent residence in the United States. On July 1, a little more than three months later, he began an internship at Memorial Hospital of DuPage County, Elmhurst, Illinois. He stayed there until June 30, 1954, when he left for Tennessee, eventually spending twelve years there before coming to Albuquerque in 1966. (Although he has never lived or practiced in Ohio, Ludwig is for some reason licensed in that state.)

While in Tennessee, Ludwig became a naturalized citizen. On June 3, 1959, adjudged by the official Justice Department examiner to be of good moral character, Ludwig told United States District Court Presiding Judge Robert L. Taylor, "I have four children and I would like to have for them a wide future." Along with eight others in the Knoxville courtroom, Ludwig was duly sworn in by the clerk of the court. He received naturalization certification number 7926316. The judge, convinced that the new citizens would do their "very dead level best to make this country a better place in which to live," adjourned the court.

It was during his stay in Knoxville that Ludwig held his first VA job. Responsible for the out-patient clinic, he says he was active in improving the treatment veterans were getting. "I was quite furious with it when I took it over," he says. "It was very unsafe, a very dirty place. I pride myself that I brought it up to better standards."

Before coming to the VA, Ludwig worked for eight years at Eastern State Hospital (now Lakeshore), a Tennessee state psychiatric facility.

People there still remember him.

"He became markedly cool to me when he found out I was Jewish," says Dr. Stanley Webster, a psychologist. Webster says Ludwig told his fellow workers that he had served in the German armed forces. When pressed, Webster adds, Ludwig amended it to "not really" in the army. He never explained further.

Ludwig was very clear about Webster, however.

"Webster?" Ludwig asked on the phone before he hung up in anger over the Bataan questions. "Webster. Oh, yes. I remember him. A Jewish doctor, a Jewish fellow. Very nice guy. One of the nicest I knew there, really."

Ludwig feels strongly that his patients at the VA not only do not lose anything by getting treated by a foreign doctor such as himself, but, on the contrary, they gain. "I don't think it has anything to do with foreign training," he says. "Medicine is international. Our needles in Germany are the same as the needles are here. I have studied more in high school and I know so many things—philosophy, history—that it would take one or two Ph.D.s to learn all of that here. That's the main issue in this respect.

"During the war, Germany was cut off from the world in a sense. We developed the V-2 rockets, missiles, and a thousand other things. But we were not in contact with the international world of medicine. We fell behind in things like anesthesiology. When I came to the United States, I realized how far behind Germany was in anesthesiology. Medicine profits most in wartime. You learn more in medicine in wartime, particularly surgery—contagious diseases and surgical medicine, predominantly.

"As a medical student, I spent time in hospitals watching operations. I saw more things in wartime than in peacetime. You're just dealing with unusual conditions that are only found in emergency rooms here in the states. When I look around here, there are mostly European teachers in psychiatry in this country. They must know their work. Europeans have done a lot. At the university where I studied, electroshock treatment was developed there.

"When I make a diagnosis, we have a manual to go by. It's all set up. There's no way of making mistakes. Ethnic diagnosis? I think someone's pulling you by the hair. I think that's ridiculous. If you take a fellow from the Bronx or Iowa, of course you have a difference in opinion. They see people differently, they have a different way of seeing things. In diagnosing someone, a good judgment is more important than anything else. You have to know the basics of what you're dealing with. You have to know all the factors involved.

"I'm amused by a lot of things here. People whittle splinters from small wood. This tendency we don't have in Europe. I have nothing to hide."

There is a story that patients at the Albuquerque VA tell one another. It is brief, and the patients shake their heads at the telling.

It seems that an old woman would daily come by the wards, bringing bouquets of flowers to place in the rooms. The flowers were cut from her garden, and the old woman brought them voluntarily to cheer up the men in their convalescences.

Once, the story goes, VA administrators asked her not to return. Her homegrown flowers, they said, had become a health hazard. So the old woman stayed away for awhile. Shortly, the flowers began to reappear on the wards again. The patients were pleased with this. The woman, despite the VA, had returned.

"She still comes here," they tell each other.

General, a man is quite expendable. He can fly and
he can kill. But he has one defect: He can think.
   —*Bertolt Brecht*

If you can't believe the veteran who fought the war
and was wounded in the war, who can you believe?
         —*From* Born on the Fourth of July
         by Ron Kovic, paraplegic Vietnam
         veteran, ex-marine, born on the
         fourth of July

IO

THE AWAKENING OF AMERICA

Doug Roberson remembers exactly his arrival back in the
United States after completing three tours of duty.

"I landed at Treasure Island in San Francisco at seven-thirty
in the morning, July 7. And I was out. We got to the airport 'round
dinnertime. Everybody else wanted to take a plane home. I said
nope. I said, 'I been in Vietnam three years and eleven months
and twenty-seven days.' I said, 'I'm goin' right down that road
there and I'm goin' catch me a Greyhound bus. And I want the
slowest one that goes across this country because I'm goin' see
what I fought for.'

"And I rode the bus all the way home."

It is hot and humid—midsummer Alabama hot and humid—
and the molten night air surrounds the muffled *zzz*ing cadences
of an insect jug band like a Mule brand work glove with a thousand holes worn into it.

Inside the home of Doug and Juanita Roberson and their girl
Tammy and boy Jerry, which stands on top of a barely negotiable

clay hillside a couple miles from the community's busy combination minimart and Shell filling station, the flies have seriously
breached the tired defenses.

Doug, a trucker on and off for eleven years and currently a
logging truck mechanic, is from Gadsden, some forty miles away
through some of the gentlest curves and greenest and best-main-
tained countryside in the Southeast. Juanita, up and around again
after giving birth to baby Chris, is from Blountsville, where the
Robersons now live within the town limits.

"I'd say the population runs from seven hundred to a thousand
people," Doug remarks.

Doug, thirty-four, is a sharp-faced man with a silky rolling
pompadour, who single-handedly keeps the local Winston distrib-
utor in business. He is wearing a white T-shirt, white sweat socks
encased in mud-caked work shoes, and heavy-duty pants of un-
certain color. Underneath the trousers, a metal brace supports his
right leg. The other one has a shrapnel wound.

He hadn't yet acquired the bulky device when he rolled across
America on that journey coming home, though he had already
paid a hefty down payment on it back in Southeast Asia.

"Well, I went through four demonstrations during the trip," he
says, "and I've asked myself for the last twelve years why in the
hell did I fight for this country? Because they don't care nuthin'
about us anyway.

"Way I look at it, there's your World War I veteran. They was
welcomed home with open arms. World War II veterans. Even the
poor old Korean veterans. They was welcomed home. The Vietnam veteran? You know any state anywhere in this world, and a
Vietnam veteran, where he's employable, wantin' a job? They spit
on him. Discriminated against.

"The government has turned their back against that war. Instead of just turning their back on the war, they've turned their
back on everybody that was in that war. And they don't even want
to be reminded of it.

"And that's why they just lettin' things walk by. And it'll go on.
'Til we jump into somethin' else or there's somebody else to throw
the blame at, they're goin' throw it at the Vietnam veteran.

"Even if he runs for president, people goin' look down their nose at him and still goin' say he was in Vietnam. To be honest with you, I lost my respect for this country, especially California —Berkeley. In September 1966, we raided a North Vietnamese hospital. And we got twenty-eight prisoners out of it, just hurtin'. And then we got six six-bys of blood donated to North Vietnam by Berkeley University College of Berkeley, California."

Roberson stops to light another Winston from the stack of cigarette packages on a nearby side table. He tosses the finished butt into a glass cigarette stand. Because his features look more as if they belong to an older man, talk of Vietnam seems odd. Doug Roberson, a casual observer would guess, should be talking of Okinawa, perhaps, or Pusan and the thirty-eighth parallel.

But he speaks of Vietnam now, quietly, and a furrow knits his brow and, yes, tears are in his eyes.

"Alan's dead," Roberson says with a thicker drawl than before. "He got killed 'bout four months later. He tore his stripes off his shirt. Give 'em his ID card and told 'em to send me home, shoot me, 'cause I'm not fighting for a damn country that gives the enemy blood for them to kill us.

"He was my buddy.

"Oh, a bunch of government officials, they come over there and all this sorta good stuff and they told us that they was goin' look into it and all this other good trash.

"They never looked into it."

Roberson, a Bronze and Silver Star recipient, served under General Walt in the Fourth Reconnaissance group, a marine unit similar to the army's elite Green Berets. He returned home with most of his left lung gone, damaged and painful knees, a history of malaria, and eleven bouts of pneumonia. The way he tells it, he'd almost rather be back in the bush instead of at the mercy of the VA.

He visits the Birmingham VA twice a year.

"Here's a joke," he says. "I go back every six months. I walk in there and he says, 'Well, you still alive?' He listens to my chest, takes my pulse and my temperature, and he asks me if my medicine's doin' alright. Then he says, 'If you ever get a chance now, cut down on that smoking.' And that's it. That's what I go down every six months for.

"But here's the catch. I got my medicine back and I carry a bottle to the shop and I keep one here. I take it every four hours. I took it at eight o'clock. By nine-thirty I was as red as you could believe. By one-thirty, I was laying here on this couch, and I didn't know I was in this world. I don't even remember drivin' home.

"My wife carried me down to the VA hospital. I had a drug reaction from the medicine I had got from the VA hospital. And the doctor told me that it wasn't even my medicine. It was my prescription, but it wasn't my medicine. You know what they said about it? 'It won't happen again.'

"But he also told me if I hadn't got there, I would've died. My muscles were cramping, and it was gettin' up to my heart. I asked him what it was. He said it was for people who got multiple sclerosis. They're bedridden, they can't even move their hands. 'We give 'em that medicine so their muscles would draw up and make them work.' That's what they sent me. And all they got to say about it was 'Sorry 'bout that.'

"He wanted them bottles back. I said, 'No, doc. I want them pills, 'cause I don't know how or when or where, but you people are goin' pay for that mistake. Just you bein' sorry—I don't go that game no more.' "

Roberson, service-connected for his lungs and knees, says, "If you want to see something sickening, go down to the emergency room [at Birmingham] and you'll see them bring somebody up from the ambulance. He might have had a heart attack. He'll lay there in that hall until his number's called, or his name comes up, or they get his records. Down here, they got to have them records before they touch you.

"My daddy went there. He was a hundred-percent-disabled veteran when he died. That's one reason I went into military service, 'cause my daddy was dyin' at the VA hospital, drawin' nineteen dollars a month, unable to work, and he was service-connected. My mother was takin' laundry in and washin' clothes, and cleanin' houses. Puttin' me through school.

"The day I turned my seventeenth birthday, I joined the service. I quit school and joined that service for one reason: to lighten the burden off my momma so I could help her. In 1964, they give my daddy his hundred-percent disability. Now here comes the catch: He died in 1965."

Roberson says VA doctors in Mississippi said he was so sick they wondered why he was working. When Roberson told them he was only getting 30 percent disability payments, they understood.

"They didn't even ask. He said, 'You're from the Alabama VA. That explains the whole situation.' "

But not entirely. After finishing at the top of his trade-school class with honors in diesel mechanics, Doug found his medical problems interfering with his ability to earn a decent living.

"Right now, there ain't nothin' rolling on wheels that I can't fix," he says. "But if I do diesel work, the next morning when I get up, I'm spittin' blood. And I have to keep doin' it. I'll always keep doin' it. I'll always feed my family. But they said down yonder, the reason I spit up that blood was because when they operated on my lung and sewed it back up, the stitches, instead of dissolvin', they just went inside my lung. The medicine don't help. But when I go down to that VA hospital, and I tell 'em I'm still spittin' up blood, they look at me like I'm that wall fixin' to move."

Roberson gets a total of $221 a month from the VA. He doesn't qualify for the GI bill and a higher-paying job because he cannot pass the physical because of the wounds he received in combat. At work, they offered him a 6¢-per-hour pay increase, while a much less experienced, but physically healthier, young boy "right next to me" got a 64¢ raise.

"They just don't want me with most of my lung gone. Don't matter that I'm the best mechanic they can get. I read all the books. I know how to fix them suckers. There's just enough wrong with me to stop me from gettin' a decent-paying job. I go to work at seven-thirty in the morning, and I get off at five. Thirty minutes off for lunch. I work five and a half days a week. I get paid no overtime. I work fifty-five to sixty hours a week.

"There's some weeks I come home seven-thirty, eight o'clock at night. Some Saturdays I work all day. Like July Fourth. Boss cussed us out 'cause we didn't work on the Fourth. That's the kind of jobs I have to take 'cause of the lung and a stinkin' piece of steel down there."

Roberson, whose hair turned silver-gray after he slept in Agent Orange powder that fell off trees "like cotton," does not expect to live past fifty. His hair has returned to its original black color—"The doctor said it was a chemical reaction to the Agent Orange," he says. "I never could understand what happened"—but he's still concerned about his future.

"Every time I go to the VA, I see a different doctor. It's never the same one, and each visit they tell me something else about my lung. Every time I turn around, I got something else wrong with me. I just set there and listen to 'em. It goes in one ear and out the other. I seen 'em so much, I don't let it bother me."

Doug stops for a moment to reprimand eight-year-old Jerry for turning on the TV set.

"My attitude toward life is zilch. That's what I got from Vietnam," he says. "In other words, I got the goals to make them"—he nods toward his wife and children—"a living. But as far as me, hell, if I wasn't married, nobody would see me. I'd get away from everybody.

"I seen so much death. My own father's death. A tear come into my eyes. I seen so much that my insides are just dead-hardened. To me a dead body, even if it's one of my kids, is dead. It's not mine anymore. I've just seen so much stinkin' death. There's a lot of us come back like that.

"One psychiatrist down here at Birmingham, she told me, 'You're among the few people, the best profession you could go in is a hired killer.' I told her, 'Honey, that depends on how much money it pays.' She said, 'Why?' I told her, ' 'Cause I got a wife and two kids at home and I can't get a decent-payin' job, and if it pays more than what I'm makin' now, then I'll take it.'

"She says, 'That's what I'm gettin' at. You'd do anything.' I said, 'That's right.' "

The nighttime has matured now outside the Robersons' home. The insects have quieted, but the oppressive heat still hangs over the living room. Doug is down to his last three packs of Winstons. He reaches under a small coffee table and brings out a red picture album. He opens it to the marine certificates he has earned. He long ago threw away his Bronze and Silver Stars. A few pages farther along are color photos of daughter Tammy's county champion softball team, the Devils.

He looks up from the memories. Across the way, hanging on the wood veneer wall, is a colorful commercially produced rug of the Last Supper.

"I got a boy who's eight years old," Doug Roberson says. "I was born and raised in this country and I was raised up by a veteran that believed that I've got the right as any man black, white, pink, or purple to help himself.

"But I've got one obligation. Every male in this country has got one obligation. He's got a military obligation ahead of him. His father had it, and he done it. He has got an obligation to serve this country. My boy's eight years old now. When he gets out of high school, if he don't want to go to college, he'll go in the service.

"So my boy's got that obligation. I hope," Doug Roberson says into the humid air, "he goes into the Marine Corps. And I hope he's good enough to make Fourth Recon. 'Cause I loved it."

Jonathan Steinberg, the busy chief counsel to Senator Cranston's Veterans' Affairs Committee, was being put on the spot by his boss. Cranston, sitting on a museum-piece chair in his cavernous office hidden away in the off-limits recesses of the Capitol, turned to Steinberg and asked him to rate the VA.

"On a scale of one to a hundred?" Steinberg replied, playing for a little more time.

Cranston nodded, a trace of a smile emerging on his thin, tanned face.

"I'd give it a seventy," Steinberg offered.

Cranston wasn't finished. "What about county hospitals?"

"Sixty-five."

"Voluntary [private] hospitals?"

"Seventy-five."

The numbers seemed to satisfy Cranston. They also appeared to support his contention, falling as they did within a few percentage points of one another, that the VA, despite all the uproar over its ability to deliver care, should remain the sole provider of that care. "The VA should not be assimilated into a bigger system," Cranston says, referring to suggestions that veterans might be better served if the VA became part of some kind of national health-care program. "It's already big enough. I believe in diversity. Combat vets couldn't be taken care of properly in a county hospital. And what if there's another war? There wouldn't be any facilities for the veterans.

"We have obligations. The system should be ready for their special needs. When people volunteer for the army, they consider the benefits. We have to remember that."

The debate over the future of the VA basically boils down to the one enunciated by Senator Cranston: Should the VA remain a separate, in effect specialized, entity, or should it move physically, administratively, and financially into the mainstream of medical care in this country? More specifically, the question can be posed, Why should the VA remain separate? What benefits do its consumers, the veterans, gain from that kind of arrangement?

From the evidence, the quick answer is, not much. If it's special care the veteran is seeking—attention to war wounds, for example—then it is clear the VA offers no more expertise than the local community hospital. Returning Vietnam vets have for over a decade loudly pointed out the lack of programs geared to their needs. And residents in training, who presumably are learning something about injuries unique to the veteran, by and large never return to the VA to utilize what they've learned once their training is over.

And, in the area of care for the aging, where the numbers of veterans are expected to increase dramatically in the next few years, the VA is playing catch-up.

Even in intangible areas, such as the camaraderie among fellow soldiers that many veterans' organizations cite as crucial for maintaining the VA as is, the argument is weakened by the fact that America's recent wars, at least, have not been very popular. And no one, especially those who fought them, is very much interested in recalling the details of the action overseas.

But the more complex answer to the question of the VA's existence must consider all of that, and more. If the veterans don't gain anything they couldn't get elsewhere—and remember, the overwhelming majority of veterans in this country do not seek VA medical care at all, and never have—then who does stand to gain from maintaining the present system?

Twenty billion dollars can go a long way to ensure the retention of the VA. But the fact is that some three-quarters of that money is used to pay for a variety of benefits—education, monthly compensation, housing, and the like—which do not necessitate a VA per se. The checks do not have to be written from the building on Vermont Avenue in Washington, D.C.

The Department of Medicine and Surgery—the hospitals—is another matter. The VA is sort of a transition mechanism between war and the return to civilian life. To the extent that it fails in that mission, it has failed in society's promise to provide the help that is needed once service to the country has been rendered. Virtually no other country has anything like the VA. There are two major reasons for that. One, very few countries try to maintain the high visibility of the veteran day in and day out to the extent that we do in this country. VA hospitals provide one means for accomplishing that.

Second, in few other countries is medical care, for veterans and nonveterans, so restricted by the ability to pay. Thus, elsewhere, no artificial financial barriers are placed in the way of veterans, since any citizen of the country is entitled to free or low-cost care. We too often forget in the United States that health care is a right, not a privilege. And it is the veteran's right, no less than the nonveteran's, to be provided with quality treatment without consideration for the number of bills in his wallet.

Proposed alternatives to the present setup have been varied. There are those who suggest paying the raw recruit a lump sum when he or she enters service. On leaving, the monies can be used in whatever way the veteran sees fit. The proponents of this plan, particularly economist Cotton Lindsay, point out that the families of soldiers killed in battle, who ordinarily would never get many of the benefits accruing to a live veteran, would thereby be served more equitably. Others recommend the issuance of chits to all discharged veterans, which would enable them to choose the source of medical care. Insurance underwritten by the U.S. government would then pay the bills, whether the provider was in the private sector or in a government facility.

Although the major veterans' organizations have loudly voiced their support of the continuation of the present system, no one has attempted any kind of systematic effort to determine the thoughts of individual consumers themselves. In California, which has the largest concentration of veterans in the country, there is a move at least to involve the patients in some mechanism for input into the VA system.

"I'm not really enamored with the idea of veterans being perpetuated in institutions exclusively for veterans," says Ron Bitzer, the director of the Center for Veterans' Rights in Los Angeles. "I would favor the folding in of veterans' programs into a larger system of health care that would distribute resources over a broader segment of the population besides just veterans." Bitzer, instrumental in trying to get patient advocates placed in the VA hospitals of southern California, points out that it might even be better psychologically for veterans to be phased in to the civilian population. "But veterans need to be part of the decision-making," he says.

Sometimes, that is even more difficult than it might seem.

"The VA is just as insensitive as the criminal justice system," says Eldson McGhee. McGhee should know. He is a Vietnam veteran, honorably discharged with a fistful of medals from the army. Since 1972, he has been in the federal penitentiary in Atlanta. He is serving a life sentence plus five years for aiding and abetting other individuals in a bank robbery. The court agreed that McGhee did not commit the crime itself. It also agreed to a much lighter sentence for one of the actual participants who turned state's evidence. McGhee, eligible for parole in 1982, maintains he is innocent.

The Atlanta pen is one of the most notorious in the system. It bristles with guard towers, high walls, and chain-link fencing with barbed wire strung across the top. A guard in a tower at the front entrance instructs all visitors to listen to a two-minute tape recording of the institution's rules and regulations.

McGhee is waiting in the interview room. There are some half dozen broken pay phones lining the peeling walls. Somewhat beside the point, one sign warns: "Do not remove receiver off hook unless instructed by telephone coordinator." Another reads: "Do not ask to see another inmate's phone card. It is not allowed."

There are a lot of "do nots" all over the place. The most obvious is the barred door with a small reinforced glass window. Someone comes over and locks the door to the interview room.

McGhee is dressed in tan slacks and a neatly pressed army fatigue shirt. His combed-back Afro is accented by a shock of gray hair on the right side of his head. He is intelligent and quiet-spoken. He is also one of the 130,000 Vietnam Era veterans in prison in this country—comprising an incredible 25–30 percent of all adult males serving jail sentences.

"The VA, basically, looks at incarcerated veterans as a low priority," McGhee, thirty-three and married, says. "There is a lack of interest on the part of the VA."

The VA, he says, does not come out on a regular basis to the pen, even though there are a large number of veterans there. What the VA does is set up an appointment for the vet to go see the VA representative. When McGhee missed an appointment recently for a disability examination, the VA disregarded his explanation that he was being forcibly detained.

"They don't make arrangements," he says. "When I wrote them and explained the situation, they said I would have to get my claim re-evaluated—get all the documents, start all over again." While in prison, McGhee has earned a B.A. degree from Mercer College and has become a sort of one-man clearinghouse for veteran inmates with problems. He says the VA could be of real help in the rehabilitation of many of the prisoners, if only it cared.

"A lot of veterans reject the VA because it doesn't fit their problems," he says. "The VA never takes into consideration that if they're going to formulate a policy, they'd better consult the veteran, see what he needs. The VA is insensitive. It's not in touch. We don't want welfare. We just want support for other veterans.

"The VA is a lot of red tape. It doesn't deviate from its way of doing things. It is bad news for lots of guys in this institution."

Jack Whitehouse, a former California cop who contracted

polio, also knows about institutions. A paratrooper in Korea and now a college criminal justice instructor and author, Whitehouse has spent a total of eleven years in a VA hospital. He is surrounded there by life-support systems. He is completely motionless except for his mouth, face, and head. In order to turn the pages of a book raised on an easel in front of him, he must use a wooden, clawlike stick clasped in his teeth.

In 1969, he was threatened by the staff with electroshock treatment because he complained about conditions on the ward.

"In reality, you suffer a double imprisonment here," he says. "You're imprisoned in an institution and you're imprisoned in a useless body. I think it's worse than being in Chino [state pen] or someplace like that. One of my friends went out to Chino and I asked him to measure the space allocated to each guy up there, and the amenities. It was better at Chino than it is here.

"You can't assume the VA operates logically," he sadly concludes.

"There's still hope among veterans," McGhee, three thousand miles away in another federal institution, says. "We're hoping to build on that before it's too late. Veterans are still young enough to have hope. But the VA is taking hope away from them. Our benefits are running out. You put a veteran back on the streets, and he's free as far as the penal system is concerned. But he's not really free if he doesn't have any marketable skills. What is he going to do then?"

The answer goes beyond veterans, beyond jails. It strikes at the very foundations of our ideas about government, about ourselves. The answer dwells not so much on whether to dismantle the VA system. It is more serious than that. The response we must adopt will have to address the changes in the attitudes we have toward people who are poor, who are suffering.

The answer must be responsive to those who have served their country and to those who "only" live and earn a living here. Medical care must be free or low-cost and of high quality. If there are special groups—children, diabetics, paraplegics, veterans, whoever—who need special and specialized care, they should get it. And where they get it should be left up to them in this pluralistic society. If the VA is as good as it says it is, veterans free to choose will be demanding VA services. If it is not, well . . .

Veterans generally do not vote as a bloc. That is one reason they can be ignored. That, and the fact that they grow old and die, and a new generation, with its own concerns, comes to take their place. It's the old college syndrome: With students passing by every four years or so, administration can wait out the demands of the freshmen, knowing full well that time and, perhaps, a new perspective will eventually dull their thrust. Yet, groups like the VFW, the American Legion, the DAV—along with Swords to Plowshares, the National Association of Concerned Veterans, Flower of the Dragon, and the rest of the new breed—can provide some lobbying pressure. It is easy to find oneself on the side of the Legionnaires: If more money is needed, then get more money. The VA, like all social welfare programs in their broadest sense in this country, always gets its budget cut first. That, too, tells us something about ourselves, and whom we honor.

But there is an important caveat to all that. When all is said and done, the blame cannot be put entirely on the VA. Congress, our elected representatives, must also share that burden. And money alone will by no means solve all the problems. It didn't when the sums were abundant, and it won't in the future. (In 1977, VA health care was roughly 25 percent of *all* federal health outlays, excluding Medicare and Medicaid.)

But a strong, involved advocacy would, one that includes the patients themselves. That is basic. For when you look around and pick out the most prosperous of the federal agencies, you notice very quickly a dedicated self-interest group, with lots of money, plenty of top-notch facilities, and high-quality staff. It is no coincidence that in the Department of Defense, if funds and programs and commitment are needed, they are always delivered. Remember: It is the DOD that makes the VA necessary in the first place.

Eldson McGhee thinks it's not too late yet to turn things around. But he issues a warning.

"Society itself has got to wake up to what's happening," he says. "If we don't start having some sensitivity toward veterans when they come back, you know, we might be creating a monster. You can't keep training people in the use of destruction and expect them to come back into this country and be the prime of citizenship.

"The next veteran may not be as patient, as tolerant, as the veteran you have now. So you better have a piece of the system for the vet when he does come back. And that has just got to include the VA."

The hour interview is over, and the jailer comes to take the prisoner back to his cell. There is some brief good-natured banter as the two start to leave. McGhee turns. He has one more thing to say.

"America will have to wake up," McGhee says quietly.

And then he is led back into the bowels of the Atlanta Federal Penitentiary.

7/81